KT-547-217

ACUPRESSURE

Eliana Harvey & Mary Jane Oatley

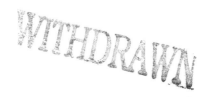
Headway • Hodder & Stoughton

The author and publishers would like to thank Christina Jansen for the cover photograph, Roddy Paine for the commissioned photographs, The University of California Press for the photograph on page 14, Hulton-Deutsch for the photograph on page 16, and Peters and Zabransky for the line drawings.

British Library Cataloguing in Publication Data

Harvey, Eliana
  Acupressure. – (Headway Lifeguides)
  I. Title II. Series
  615.822

ISBN 0 340 611065

First published 1994
Impression number 10 9 8 7 6 5 4 3 2 1
Year   1998 1997 1996 1995 1994

Typeset by Wearset, Boldon, Tyne and Wear.
Printed in Great Britain for Hodder & Stoughton Educational, a division of Hodder Headline Plc, 338 Euston Road, London NW1 3BH by St Edmundsbury Press Ltd.

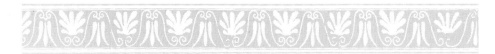

CONTENTS

Standard meridian abbreviations used in this book

CV	Conception Vessel
GV	Governing Vessel
Lu	Lung
Co	Colon
Sp	Spleen
St	Stomach
P	Pericardium
Th	Triple heater
H	Heart
Si	Small intestine
Li	Large intestine
Lv	Liver
Gb	Gall-bladder
Ki	Kidneys
Bl	Bladder

INTRODUCTION

What is Acupressure?

Acupressure is a very ancient healing therapy that has its origins in early China. It is based on a belief fundamental to all branches of oriental medicine – namely that there exists a network of energy lines throughout the body called 'meridians'. These energy meridians are the conduit for the vital force, or 'qi' (pronounced 'chee') which flows through the body, rather like the current of a river. This qi, or life force, can become blocked, or stagnant, as can water whose flow has been interrupted, and this is what happens when we become unwell. Our health and well-being are dependent on the harmonious flow of qi in our body, nourishing and balancing us at cellular level. Qi can be brought into balance through activating the acupoints, small vortices of energy distributed along the whole length of each meridian flow.

In acupressure, the therapist uses hands and fingertips to activate the points found along the meridians, which makes it different from acupuncture where needles are used. It is necessary to touch only a couple of points to alleviate particular aches and pains for first aid or relaxation (relief from stress). But, ideally, one has a full body treatment in which a therapist or friend uses a combination of points to achieve a profounder effect. This rebalancing of the body is partly achieved through different qualities of touch and pressure, using hands, fingertips and, in the case of Shiatsu, elbows and feet.

There are several forms of acupressure, which, together with acupuncture, use the same meridian system and acupoints, all drawing their knowledge from ancient oriental medical and philosophical systems. Some of these systems need to be undertaken by professionals, others you can try yourself.

Systems delivered by professionals

Of these forms, Shiatsu from Japan is probably the most widely known. The client is treated at floor level on a thin mattress 'futon' and the practitioner uses a fair amount of body weight and pressure from fingers, thumbs, hands, elbows and, sometimes, feet. In addition to its benefits, Shiatsu is particularly useful for relieving deep muscular tension.

Other forms of acupressure that are Japanese in origin are Jin Shin Jyutsu and Jin Shin Do. These treatments are usually given on a massage table or low couch. Jin Shin Jyutsu uses very light touch and the emphasis is more on spiritual and emotional rebalancing as a starting point for healing. Jin Shin Do works with firmer pressure and aims to release body 'armouring'. It would be considered useful in preventive medicine, as well as dealing with particular conditions. Shen Tao has links with Jin Shin Do and Jin Shin Jyutsu, but has as its basis Chinese medicine and Taoist philosophy.

These three forms use both hands, so a circuit of energy is created between the practitioner and the client. This may involve pressure, rubbing, stroking, tapping and vibration. These forms also have the ability to work on more subtle levels of the body. They are suited to physical problems, but at deeper levels become very gentle healing systems for mind, emotions and spirit and are effective for those who need to be helped with great compassion. Shen Tao is also appropriate for people who meditate and have begun to work on a spiritual path.

Systems to try yourself

There are also many kinds of oriental self-massage which include working on the meridians and acupoints. There are effective methods of self-treatment offered by Do In and G-Jo, both Japanese, using single points or areas on a meridian line for first aid, pain relief and preventive care.

Shen Tao and Jin Shin Do can also offer simple self-care treatments; they use both hands. The *mudras* (a word originally meaning the gestures of Buddha's hands) of 'harmonisation' also use both hands and are mainly for spiritual and emotional healing. It is quite possible to learn how to give yourself or your family effective treatment by means of clear instructions and diagrams.

Suggestions for books currently in print are given in Further Reading, at the end of this book. Many of the books on acupressure are written by acupuncturists who sometimes substitute finger pressure for use of needles, especially when dealing with children or people who are afraid of needles.

What is Qi?

The quality of our vital energy is determined by the state of health of our parents at the time of our conception. The younger and healthier the parents, the more the possibility that the child will have a strong constitution and an abundance of qi. But if the parents are weak (through illness, poor constitution or undernourishment), or are older, the quality of qi of the child will be less vital. The quality of qi is also much influenced by nourishment from the mother's kidneys during pregnancy. Therefore, it is important that the mother has a good diet with plenty of vitamins and minerals, and that she tries to have regular exercise during pregnancy. It is also important to stop smoking and not to drink alcohol during pregnancy, and to take ample rest.

Thus, our basic constitutional qi is largely influenced by the state of health and age of our parents and it is difficult to change the quality of this qi. After we are born the quality of qi can, however, be influenced by the quality of our diet, how we digest it, how we breathe, our state of mind, our emotions, how much exercise we take and whether we can create a balance between work and times of relaxation. Breathing exercises and forms such as Qi Gong, Tai Chi and Yoga are extremely helpful for vitalising the being, and supplementing the qi. Practitioners of Jin Shin Jyutsu and Shen Tao energise their hands and fingers by using the breath and visualisation to channel the qi; yoga practitioners know this energy as Prana, and practitioners of Japanese martial arts know it as Ki.

There are a number of exercises to channel this energy to increase one's store of qi, which are especially important before self-treatment.

Exercise

a) Sit in a comfortable position with your spine straight but not stiff, shoulders relaxed, palms face up, hands resting on knees. Mentally create a tube or pathway from an opening at the crown of the head down to the heart, then branching out to the shoulders, arms and hands.

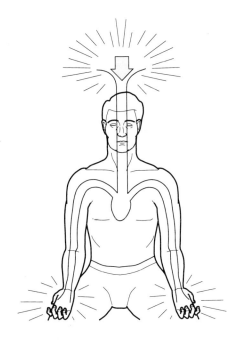

As you breathe *in* visualise sparkling silvery or golden light flowing to the heart; on the *out* breath, direct this energy up the shoulders and down to the fingers. After a moment or two, warmth and tingling is usually felt.

b) This exercise is often made more effective for beginners by taking each arm in turn and moving the qi from heart to fingertips for a few moments, with the opposite hand about two inches away from the body. Repeat the exercise using the other hand.

c) When the hands feel energised, experiment by holding the palms almost together and then draw them backwards gently until they are about three feet apart. Keep moving them back and forth and notice not only the sensations in the hands and fingers but also the quality of energy in the space between the hands. The space may feel 'alive' and you may begin to play with the energy ball you have created.

Without the channeling of qi much more pressure will be needed when an acupoint is activated, but if the qi is directed through the fingertips, rather like little lasers, a light touch is more effective, as it is the qi that does the work.

None of this is surprising when we remember that we are made up of pure energy particles, simply compacted and differentiated for various functions. The Chinese were aware of this in their own way, more than 5000 years ago.

Yin and Yang

Our life force, or qi, is composed of two types of energy, namely Yin and Yang. In oriental philosophy everything consists of yin and yang. Yin is considered the receptive, and yang the active, energy.

A short list of yin and yang qualities shows the different aspects that fall under one or the other category.

YIN	*YANG*
receptive	active
negative	positive
dark, hidden	light, exposed
female	male
inside	outside
depleted	overstimulated
introvert	extrovert
below	above
contraction	expansion
cold	hot

From an oriental point of view, everything is either yin or yang. It is possible to look at anything in life and discover its yin and its yang aspect. A tree, for example, has its yang aspect on the outside, the bark, and its yin aspect underneath the bark, the trunk. Going a step further, it has its trunk as an exposed part, which is yang, and its roots as a hidden part, which is yin. The roots are of great importance to the tree, as these unexposed roots supply the tree with energy and its life. It is the same with people and animals. The unexposed parts, the organs, blood, lymph, bone marrow, supply us with energy and are needed to keep us healthy and alive.

Some other examples of yin and yang are the positive and negative terminals of a battery; the different seasons (summer is yang, winter is yin, spring is yang, autumn is yin); ice is yin, water is yang; a dark room is yin, a well-lit room is yang.

The outside of our body is yang, the inside is yin. Certain organs inside our body are considered yang organs (small intestine, gall-bladder, bladder, colon, stomach) and others yin (heart, pericardium, liver, kidneys, lungs, spleen). Our blood is yin, but our lymphatic fluids are yang. Our brain is considered a yin organ.

Everything in life has an active or a receptive part. Every human being has a male and a female aspect; in some people the male aspect and, therefore, its active side, is more developed, while in others the female aspect, or its receptive side, is more developed. Yin and yang are opposite forces, but they complement each other at the same time, and depend on each other for existence. In an ideal situation a person would have these two aspects completely in balance and would use both sides in equal strength.

Achieving a totally balanced male and female aspect requires a lot of dedication and constant contemplation of oneself and one's life. One's constitution at birth, and many outside influences throughout life, can be great obstacles in trying to achieve this equilibrium.

Yin energy inside the body is related to storing vital energy and vital essence in some organs, such as the lungs, spleen, kidneys, liver and heart. Yang is related to transmitting and digesting food in some organs, such as the large intestine, small intestine, bladder, gall-bladder and stomach. If a person is in good health, there is a balance between the yin and yang energies. If the balance is disturbed, however (if yin is greater than yang energy or vice versa), illness arises. Imbalances can be caused through diet, lifestyle, mental and/or emotional problems.

YIN & YANG SYMBOL OF ETERNAL LAW
IN MANIFESTATION

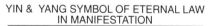

THE WAVELIKE FLOW OF YIN TO YANG AND
YANG TO YIN ACTIVATED BY QI

WHITE YANG

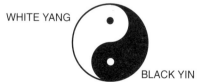

BLACK YIN

THE CONTINUOUS CIRCLE OF WHOLENESS, UNITY
CHANGE AND BALANCE
NOTHING IS WHOLLY YIN OR YANG

The Yin-Yang symbol

The list below gives typical yin and yang characteristics. If a person has more characteristics from the yin column, he or she is yin-orientated, and vice versa.

YIN	*YANG*
introvert	extrovert
quiet	lively
speaks slowly or softly	speaks fast or loudly
very silent	laughs or giggles a lot, even when speaking
well-built, overweight sluggish	thin, anorexic
very pale skin colour	reddish facial colour
dresses in dark colours	dresses in bright colours
pulse, difficult to feel and slow	pulse full, and fast

This is a short list only, but gives an idea how we are all part of yin or yang. It is also possible, and very common, to have a combination of some elements, but in every person there will always be a predominance of either yin or yang.

The qi in our body can become blocked, stagnant or empty, as can a river. Our health and well-being are dependent on the harmonious flow of qi (and the balance between yin and yang) in our body. This can be brought into balance through activating the acupoints, little vortices of energy along the meridian flow.

The meridians

The meridians are passages through which qi and blood circulate; they are not blood vessels. It is thought that there are fourteen main meridians and a great number of secondary meridians. Twelve main meridians are located in pairs on the right side and the left side of the body, and two meridians are on the vertical midline of the body, one located on the front midline, the other on the midline on the back of the body.

The twelve meridians are classified in pairs and consist of six yin and six yang. Three yin meridians run from the chest to the hand and three yang from the hand to the head; three yang meridians from the head to the foot and three yin from the foot to the abdomen and chest.

In the interior each meridian is connected to one of the main organs in the body and each is named according to the organ to which it is connected. On the exterior each meridian connects with the body's surface and this is where acupoints are distributed, 361 points in total.

The following diagram shows how the meridians work in pairs and what their names are.

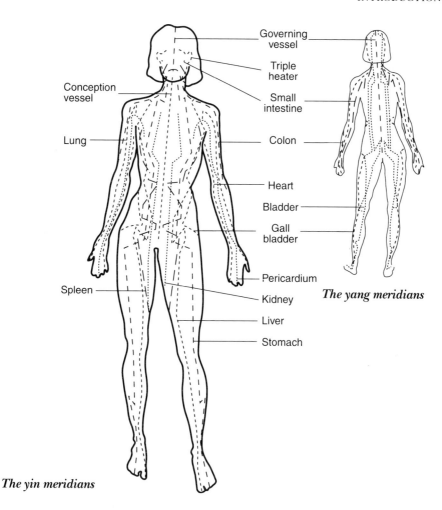

Governing vessel

Triple heater

Conception vessel

Small intestine

Lung

Colon

Heart

Bladder

Gall bladder

Pericardium

Spleen

Kidney

Liver

Stomach

The yang meridians

The yin meridians

The meridians

YIN MERIDIAN	YANG MERIDIAN
Lung	Large intestine
Triple heater	Pericardium
Heart	Small intestine
Kidney	Bladder
Spleen	Stomach
Liver	Gall-bladder

The two single meridians that run over the midline of the body are the Governing Vessel (masculine) and the Conception Vessel (feminine).

Imbalance in an organ can manifest itself in its related organ and vice versa. For example, pain along the heart meridian can indicate a heart problem, or a heart problem, such as a heart attack, can cause radiation of chest pain to the shoulder and down the whole left arm to the hand.

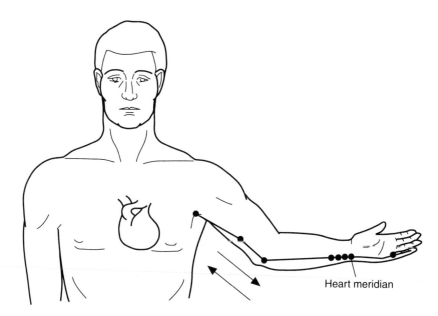

The heart meridian

If the liver is affected, for example by disease, alcohol or strong emotions, such as anger or resentment, it can cause migraines, red eyes or yellow/green skin. If any of these signs and symptoms occur it can indicate a problem with the liver.

Pain along the large intestine meridian can indicate constipation. An imbalance along the stomach meridian can show up by nausea, for example. There are many more of these examples that could be given and you will find a more detailed list in the self-treatment section.

The secondary meridians form an intricate but invisible web all over the body, similar to our network of arteries, veins and lymphatic vessels. These secondary meridians distribute qi. They can produce visible signs along their pathway, such as thread veins, skin rashes, different kinds of skin sensations, such as tingling, numbness, heat or coldness, or swollen muscles.

1

HISTORY OF ACUPRESSURE

Acupressure is the most ancient of the oriental therapies, reputed to be more than 5000 years old. It is believed that acupressure originated in India and was later spread by Buddhist monks to Central Asia, China and Egypt. The Chinese, in particular, developed the art of acupressure into an accepted and respected healing system. There are forms of Taoist massage practised today in China; these would include activation of the acupoints. It is usually firm, vigorous massage, and many of the practitioners are blind people, having been specially trained and valued for their increased sense of touch.

The Sons of Reflected Light

How the ancients came to know of the meridian acupoint system is shrouded in myth and conjecture. One of the myths of acupuncture is that soldiers in battle who were pierced by arrows (not fatally!) somehow found relief from other symptoms when the wound healed. Another delightful legend is that of extraordinary beings, called the 'Sons of Reflected Light', who arrived in China about 10,000 BC. They were seven feet tall and wore clothing of a substance never seen before. They proceeded to take the most talented practitioners of all the Arts. These beings trained them and founded schools far in advance of what was known at that time. Many forms of healing were taught. These healers were said to be highly sensitive and could see both the aura and the meridians, and the acupoints were seen as little points of light. These we now know to be points of low electrical resistance. It appears that the healers could 'see' what was wrong in the body and the energy field, and only needed to direct their qi to the person from a few feet away to make the necessary changes in the flow of the sick person's qi. It is interesting that we are now finding that certain Chinese Qi Gong practitioners seem to have regained this healing sensitivity and ability (Qi Gong is like Tai Chi).

Possibly through the centuries the healing sensitivity was lost and as healers needed to come closer to the body, they started using pressure, fingernails, pieces of pointed bone and finally gold and silver needles. At this point there seems to have been some kind of separation, with needles being the prerogative of physicians to the nobility. The intuitive natural healers with a basic medical knowledge but without needles would travel from village to village offering their services, becoming known as 'Barefoot Practitioners'.

The Nei Ching

In early times there were great differences in particular religious philosophies and methods of healing due to the vastness of China. However, in time, the Taoist philosophers in their search for the nature of man and his environment and wider spiritual concepts, came to have a unifying effect on all the diverse systems. One of the earliest writings, written about 3000 BC, is the *Yellow Emperor's Classic of Internal Medicine*, the *Nei Ching*. The first part deals with medical knowledge and the second part with the underlying spiritual aspects. A vast store of knowledge has been built up over the 5000 years since that time. Qi Gong and Tai Chi, which is having a major revival in China today and has become a major part of the medical system, are the best known forms of movement for self-healing and maintenance.

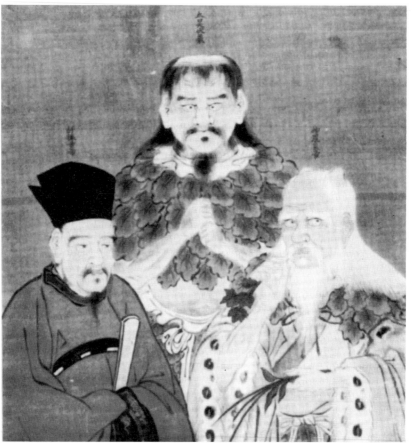

The three legendary emperors, Fu Hsi, Shen Nung and Huang Ti, who are supposed to have founded the art of healing. From a Japanese scroll by Seibi Wake, 1798. (Reproduced by kind permission of University of California Press, from The Yellow Emperor's Classic of Internal Medicine, *translated and with an introductory study by Ilza Veith, 1972, ISBN 0 520 02158 4).*

Exercise

The following exercise shows you how easy it is to see your own aura. You need to be in a well-lit room or one in which there is plenty of sunshine coming in and that has a white or light-coloured ceiling. Look up at the ceiling and bring your hands up and above your face, with your fingers spread open. Keep looking at the ceiling and slowly bring the fingers of both hands closer together until the tips of the fingers touch one another (keep fingers spread open). You are then able to see a shimmering around the fingers, which is your aura. You can continue this experiment indoors and outdoors, with plants, flowers, animals and even other people, as long as you don't look straight into the sun.

Discovery of acupoints

Through observation and experimentation in the early days, physicians developed techniques of curing illnesses and of relieving pain by pressing, with fingertips or bones on specific parts of the body, which we now call 'acupoints'. After further observation and study it was discovered that there are about 1000 acupressure points on the body. Of these, 669 are listed in a standard textbook on acupuncture which is used in modern China, written by Dr Chu Lien's *Hsin Chen Chiu Hsueth* (*Modern Acupuncture*). Of these points, the effects of many are duplicated so that 90–100 are of real importance for common ailments. Each school of acupressure or acupuncture will have developed its own repertoire of points.

Acupressure and Mao Tse-tung

The practice of acupressure and acupuncture was surrounded by myth and legend until the first half of the twentieth century, when Mao Tse-tung revived these ancient therapies and brought their practice more in line with modern understanding. However, it took another 20 years before the outside world became more aware of this method of healing. A Western journalist, James Reston, visiting China in 1971, was saved from an emergency appendix operation through acupuncture. Thereafter, a number of Western medical practitioners visited China to observe the healing effects of these therapies.

Western scientists researched the existence of meridians and acupoints as well, eventually confirming what the ancients had discovered by using sensitive electrical equipment. Dr Hiroshi Motoyama, who is a Shinto priest, scientist and acupuncturist, created a machine, a physiological recording device, capable of scientifically measuring the meridians and the chakras. Through intensive yogic exercises he became keenly aware of his own chakras. He was recognised by UNESCO in 1974 as one of the most excellent parapsychologists in the world. We now know that certain acupoints affect certain chakras.

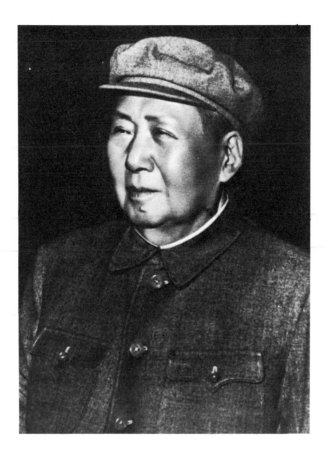

Mao Tse-tung (1893–1976)

Scientifically speaking

It is known that endorphins are released in the brain when acupoints are stimulated with pressure, needles or heat. Endorphins are neurochemicals that relieve pain. Releasing them creates a greater flow of blood and oxygen to the affected area, making the muscles relax, the pain subside and enabling healing to take place. Acupressure, through stimulating the acupoints just under the skin, inhibits pain signals sent to the brain.

For thousands of years, the Chinese have used acupressure as well as acupuncture to relieve pain, and also to ease tensions and stress and balance the whole body and its immune system. Acupressure was also used as a beauty therapy, for example to improve facial circulation, and reduce puffiness and fine lines around the eyes. Some exercises for facial treatments are given in Chapter 8.

2

ACUPRESSURE IN THE EAST AND WEST

The differences between Eastern and Western approaches

Acupressure and acupuncture, like Western antibiotics, are very effective in treating disease. However, much is still unknown about oriental medicine, how it works and why it works. As a result, the Western world sometimes has difficulty accepting the values of oriental medicine, and one often hears the phrase 'It's all in the mind'. Some people are of the opposite opinion and believe that as oriental medicine is more ancient, it is therefore more holistic and better than Western medicine. Unfortunately, this kind of attitude has the danger of turning oriental medicine into a religion rather than a medical body of science.

Oriental medicine has developed over two millenia and has been further developed as a result of continual rigorous observation and analytical thought. If Eastern and Western methods of treating disease differ profoundly, even more significant is their different philosophy and interpretation fundamental to the world we live in and the way that human beings react and interact with that world.

The diagnosis

The orientals have always had a different way of looking at the body and its ailments from the West. They look at a person as a whole and look at body, mind and emotions, all at the same time. A diagnosis is made accordingly. Therefore, if a person has an ailment or a chronic problem, an oriental physican looks at the patient's diet, lifestyle, how the patient looks (facial colour, body posture, etc.), how he talks and moves about, even how the patient is dressed and what colours he wears. The physician then makes a diagnosis and decides which organ(s) and which meridian(s) are likely to be affected. After that, the physician makes a decision whether his patient has an overstimulated system and needs sedation, or a depleted system that needs stimulation on certain acupoints.

The treatment

Oriental and Western medicines treat the body in different ways; the differences lie in their approach and their terminology. The most obvious difference is that oriental thought does not name a disease but rather describes a group of observed disharmonious patterns by naming the causes. Names are given to describe the diagnosis, such as 'Cold', 'Heat', 'Wind', 'Dampness' and even stranger to the Western ear, 'Internal Cold or Heat' or 'External Cold or Heat', 'Internal or External Wind or Dampness'. Usually a combination of these is used, so a diagnosis could be 'Internal Wind-Heat' or 'External Damp-Cold'. A diagnosis for a stroke could be 'Liver-Wind', or for psoriasis, which looks very red, 'Internal Wind-Heat'.

Western medicine looks in greater detail at some areas of the body, such as the nervous system, the endocrine system, or the circulation of blood and lymph. It seeks to discover and name a disease by a narrow focus which analyses and isolates a particular condition. From a set of symptoms a cause is sought, a disease named and, usually, a precise single medication prescribed, which seldom takes the totality of the being into account. Oriental medicine does not look at any of these areas in isolation, but will treat nervous, endocrine, or blood disorders as part of a whole imbalance. Diagnosis is made in a different way, and treatments may consist of number of complementary therapies, such as acupressure or acupuncture, heat treatment and herbs, and Qi Gong. In addition, the points used may well vary from treatment to treatment as subtle alterations are noted in the condition from week to week.

A Western physician starts by looking at a symptom and then will try to find the cause; treatment is directed more at curing the symptom. A Chinese physician, however, will look at the whole of a person, his physical, mental and emotional state, and will aim to find the cause of the problem first and treat that rather than the symptom, with the aim of clearing the symptom after treatment of the cause has taken place. Western medicine is at its most effective when dealing with acute problems, infections, surgery and problems with the skeletal structure. Oriental medicine works well with functional disorders and chronic problems.

Quite often an oriental treatment is accompanied by a prescription of herbal medicine. The use of herbs is very popular in China. Recently, the West has been taking more interest in their use, particularly to cure skin problems, such as eczema and psoriasis, where they have been found far more effective than Western remedies and treatments.

The acupoints

Each acupoint has its own Chinese name and these sound very poetic. They give an indication of the point's benefits or its location. For instance, a point located below the belly button is called 'Sea of qi' (CV6). This is a very powerful point to strengthen the body and is very useful for chronic weakness on a physical and mental level; it restores our fundamental vitality. This point is also used by the Japanese and is called the 'Hara'.

Exercise

A strengthening exercise is to hold both your hands over this point. Breathe in deeply, starting by breathing into your belly first, as if you are filling up a bottle with water, and continue breathing in to fill up your chest with breath.

Hold your breath for a few seconds and then slowly breathe out, starting by emptying the chest first and finishing with your belly. By doing this exercise for a few minutes on a daily basis, you strengthen your whole body and can dissolve sad and painful emotions.

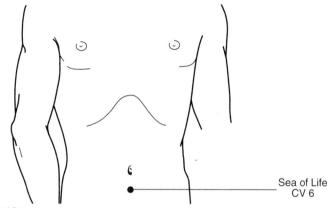

Sea of Life
CV 6

CV 6 (Sea of Life)

Another point is called 'Wind Palace' (GV 15). This point can be used for epilepsy and severe giddiness; it helps to clear the mind and stimulate the brain. Or, there is 'Mind Courtyard' (GV 24.5). This is an important point to calm the mind.

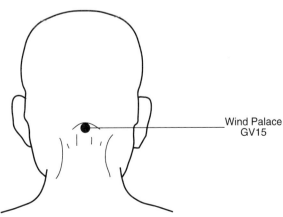

Wind Palace
GV15

GV 15 (Wind Palace)

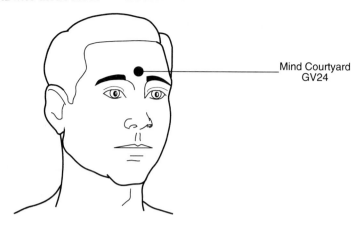

GV 24 (Mind Courtyard)

'Shoulder Convergence' (Th13) is a good point to use for pain in the upper arm, while 'Knee Gate' (Lv7) is a good point for pain in the knee, especially if on the inside of the knee.

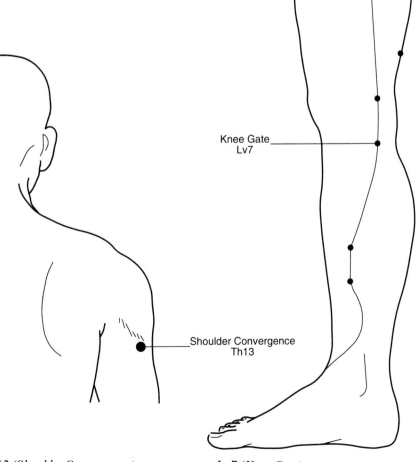

Th 13 (Shoulder Convergence)   *Lv7 (Knee Gate)*

3

THE FIVE ELEMENTS

In many traditions, life comes from the 'Original Source' into duality or polarity (yin and yang), then manifests itself in a myriad of forms of expression. In oriental philosophies, in between yin and yang and the 'many', are the 'five elements', the substance of the universe, the planet and also our bodies, defined as earth, metal, wood, fire and water; human beings are made of, reflect, and are influenced by, these five elements in the external environment. The five elements have many interactive functions, both harmonising and nurturing each other as well as regulating each other.

The nourishing cycle

Wood is good for *fire*, which leaves ashes, becoming part of the *earth* in which are found *metals* and other minerals, these liquifying or causing condensation resulting in *water*, which feeds the *trees* (wood), completing the cycle. Each is essential for the following element's existence.

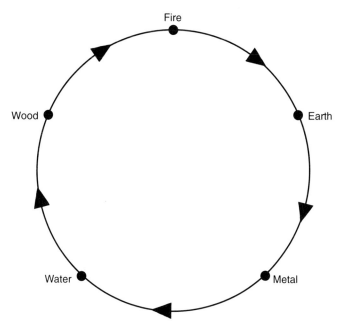

The nourishing cycle of the five elements

The regulating cycle

The regulating cycle controls excess of any element. *Metal* can pulverise *wood*; *wood* (roots) can penetrate the *earth* and break it up; *earth* can be banked to control the flow of *water*; *water* puts out *fire*; *fire* can melt *metal*.

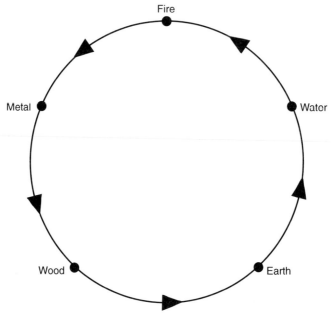

The regulating cycle of the five elements

Balance and the five elements

The five elements form a valuable map for leading a healthy life or for bringing us back into balance. Practitioners may well use the five elements philosophy as part of their diagnosis. Part of this diagnosis will include a special form of pulse-taking which reveals, among other things, what is happening in each element, along the meridian, and within the organs linked to each section of the meridian, remembering that the meridian is one continuous flow.

Each element is connected to many things internally and externally – planets, seasons, time of day, direction, climate, skin tone, senses, voice quality, emotions, internal and external anatomy, ideal foods, vegetables, fruit. On a simple level, we can see how this system works – for example, if on a summer's day we play a rigorous game of tennis, we become *red-faced*, *over-heated* and *thirsty* (all fire element aspects), so we need *liquid*, a *shower* and *relaxation* (all water element aspects) to bring us back into balance.

Example of the element 'Wood'

planet	Jupiter
season	spring
time of day	morning
direction	east
climate	wind
skin tone	green
senses	sight
voice	shouting
organ	liver
internal anatomy	muscles
external anatomy	tissues
emotion	anger
ideal food	wheat
vegetable	leek
fruit	apples
damaging drinks and foods	alcohol, coffee, dairy products, especially cheese, chocolate

So a simple overview of the five elements from a diagnostic point of view might look like this.

Fire	Wood	Water	Metal	Earth
small intestine triple heater	gall-bladder	bladder	large intestine	stomach
heart pericardium	liver	kidneys	lungs	spleen
red	green	blue/black	white	yellow
heat	wind	cold	dryness	humidity
summer	spring	winter	autumn	Indian summer
joy	anger	fear	grief	sympathy

It could be helpful to discover which element best describes us, and this way we could take preventive action, for example by looking at our diet and lifestyle. It could be even more interesting to train our perceptions by grouping our family and friends according to the element or elements they typify; this will help us to understand them in a new way.

The following descriptions provide 'thumbnail' sketches of each element type and personality.

Example of the element 'Fire'

Mrs Jones has a very volatile personality, she speaks very rapidly and never knows when to stop, her shrill laughter sounds rather hysterical sometimes; she is prone to restlessness; she likes bright colours, especially red; she possibly has circulation problems, such as varicose veins; she may eat rather fast and not digest her food too well. However, she is fun to be with, is very creative and enjoys her friends. She may have dry skin with psoriasis. She is a *fire* person.

Example of the element 'Wood'

Mr Smith is very strong-minded, rather bossy and controlling; he tends to shout, especially when angry, which he often is, as he is rather inflexible; he suffers with his digestion if he overeats; he does like rich food and a glass of wine; he has to watch his weight; he enjoys the outdoors, but high winds really irritate him; his favourite gardening job is pruning; he likes to keep the shrubs and trees in order. However, he is a very good organiser, very reliable, and always finishes what he has set out to do. He is a *wood* person.

Other signs of a wood person are: pre-menstrual tension (women), swollen breasts (women), fluid retention, scatty and aggressive, clumsy, shouting. Politicians are often inclined to be wood types especially those with deep lines around the mouth and a central line over the forehead.

Example of the element 'Metal'

Mr Grey is rather an anxious man. He is frightened of his boss and cannot stand lifts as he suffers from claustrophobia; he has a tendency to asthma and constipation and his skin is very pale and dry, except for his eczema patches which he gets when particularly stressed; he does not look very robust and is round-shouldered with a hollow chest; milk and dairy products do not seem to suit him at all, making him prone to an excess of mucus; he is sensitive and careful of others' feelings. He is a *metal* person.

Example of the element 'Earth'

Mrs Brown is a plump lady with a slightly yellowish skin tone; she enjoys cakes and sweet things, which she tends to indulge in when sad or upset, or particularly worried. She is a great worrier and cannot switch off; she did not have a very happy childhood and is over-protective of her family and others by way of compensation; she always involves herself in other people's problems; she has real difficulty with her weight and suffers from indigestion. She is an *earth* person.

Example of the element 'Water'

Mrs Black always has dark circles under her eyes; she feels the cold badly and her feet are always frozen; sometimes her complexion has a bluish tone; her hair seems to be thinning early; she complains a lot of low backache and often needs to go to the loo; she can work with feverish bursts of energy and then collapses into exhaustion; her stamina is not very good and her bones tend to fracture easily now that she is getting older. She is a *water* person.

These thumbnail sketches only show extreme examples. Within each element type, there are a wide variety of 'signs and symptoms' both positive and negative. In addition, with most people, one element will predominate, but there will be secondary aspects from one or most of the other elements.

Diet and the Five Elements

In oriental medicine it is considered that there are various foods and drinks which will damage the function of certain organs and systems if taken in excess. This connection is just beginning to come to the attention of Western medicine. The most obvious from a Western viewpoint is the effect of sugar and sweets on the spleen and pancreas which could, in time, lead to diabetes.

The lungs and colon are said to suffer from an excess of dairy products which cause a build up of mucus. In the West, it is recognised that dairy products have a worsening effect on asthma. Excess of red meat and protein damages the kidneys; in fact, any substances that cause a toxic build-up will exhaust the kidneys. The heart and pericardium are damaged by rich fatty foods and alcohol. The liver and gall-bladder are overloaded by excess fats, dairy products, especially cheese, chocolate, alcohol and coffee. In some cases, oranges affect the liver.

During the winter (yin) we should be eating yang heating foods to bring internal warmth. These are provided by root vegetables, grains and fruits of the season, for example, apples and pears. Tropical vegetables and fruits or salads, should not be eaten during winter as they are designed by nature, being yin foods, to keep us cool in the summertime (yang). If we eat lots of raw summer foods in winter we will cool and slow our digestion down, causing wind, bloating and sometimes bowel disorders.

There is an oriental saying, also known in the West, 'Eat breakfast like an emperor, lunch like a prince and supper like a pauper.' According to Chinese thinking, this is because the energy of the stomach meridian is most active first thing in the morning, and in the later evening the liver meridian needs to be left to do its work of processing the foods of the day, not to have more food thrown at it. If you habitually wake between 1 a.m. and 3 a.m., this usually confirms that too many liver-distressing substances are being consumed too late in the evening, especially cheese and alcohol. The liver and gall-bladder are also in charge of the area of the back of the neck and shoulders. So, if constant neck and shoulder tension is experienced, plus a tendency to headaches, the diet should be checked for excess consumption of liver-distressing food and drink, such as fats, alcohol, coffee and dairy products.

Never skip breakfast. It provides a good foundation for the day, both for the liver and the nervous system. If a good breakfast is not taken, this can upset the blood sugar levels. Resulting feelings of stress are often supressed by drinking the coffee, which gives a false temporary lift, but actually adds to the stress and debilitating effect on the liver. An ideal breakfast would be porridge made with organic oats, cooked with a few dates or raisins, no sugar, and a few slices of grated ginger. This provides internal warmth, slow release of energy, and is perfect for winter. Muesli with fruit and yoghurt makes a perfect summer breakfast.

The whole system benefits from the cleansing effect of a diet high in fruits and vegetables appropriate to the season of the year.

4

HOW ACUPRESSURE CAN HELP US

Stroking and soothing by the mother's hands is usually the first nurturing 'touch' experience that the child receives after birth. It is a basic and natural human impulse to heal by laying hands on the affected area to soothe it. Unfortunately, the trusting healing touch is quickly left behind in our society, especially with rising concerns about child abuse. The sad thing about this is that nurturing touch is essential for balanced emotional development and the stability of the nervous system, so it is very unfortunate that we have had to become so cautious. What happens these days is that often people have to pay to receive the healing touch – not all families are 'huggy' or able to demonstrate affection physically.

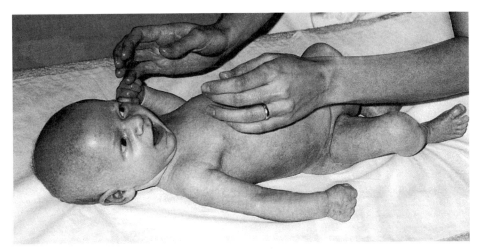

The healing touch

Focused healing touch is very powerful. Acupressure, working with simple pressure through the fingertips, can be as effective as the use of needles in acupuncture. Acupressure is particularly useful in treating the frail, the elderly, small children and those who are afraid of needles and, therefore, cannot tolerate acupuncture. Acupressure is also excellent for treating the more subtle levels of mental and emotional stress and tension caused by modern day living. Acupressure is effective with immediate illness and chronic conditions and can also help in bringing to the surface early traumatic memories in childhood which might be the root of problems being experienced today.

The qi energy that permeates the body also links into the subtle energy system and the chakra system. The knowledge and significance of these subtle energy systems has been held and developed in the East and in Buddist monasteries for many centuries.

The subtle energy bodies and the chakras

Acupressure is closely linked to our subtle energy system and chakra system. The chakras directly influence the personality, glandular system and the organs of the body.

Our body is surrounded by an aura or energy field (an exercise to see part of one's aura is given in Chapter 1). Another way of showing the aura is with Kirlian or, high voltage, photography. This technique was developed in Russia by Semyon Kirlian in 1940 and shows an energy emission around a person or an object. Certain information about a person's physical, mental and emotional condition can be concluded from these photographs, and this can be used diagnostically.

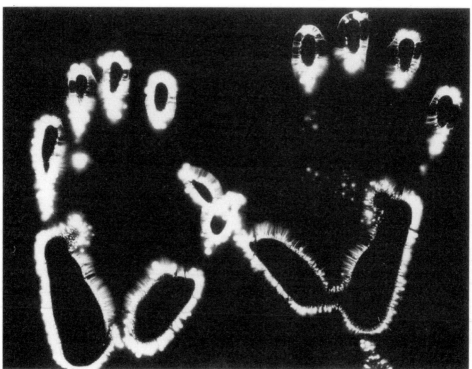

This Kirlian photograph clearly shows the energy field around the hands

The physical body is associated with 'consciousness'. The aura surrounding the physical body consists of different layers. The physical body is first surrounded by a thin layer called the 'etheric body', which connects it to its aura. The aura also consists of an 'astral body', which is associated with emotions and feelings, and a 'mental body', which is associated with thoughts and our mental state.

These three bodies, the physical, astral and mental, represent our personality. Each of the three bodies has its own corresponding 'etheric-double', an energy field that links the three bodies to one another and keeps them alive. Each body has its own system of energy channels and each etheric-double has its own system of energy centres or chakras.

The chakras

There are seven major chakras, the basic, sacral, solar plexus, heart, throat, brow and crown chakras. Furthermore, there are 21 minor chakras, located at different points in the physical body.

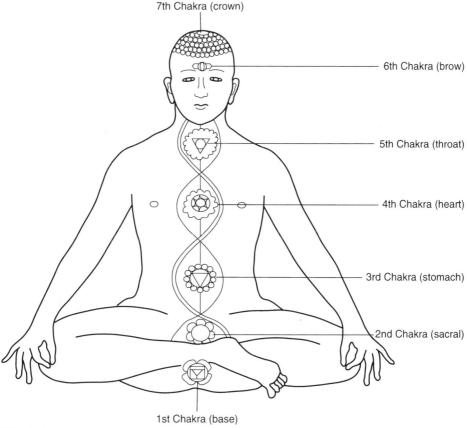

The chakra system

The name 'chakra', translated from Sanskrit, means 'wheel'. Some people who can see the chakras perceive these centres as rotating wheels or vortices of light.

The first or base chakra

The base chakra is in the area of the coccyx and is seen as a wheel of red light. This chakra controls the kidneys and the genito-urinary system. It has a slow, heavy vibration and a warm energy. The vibration releases toxins, builds up red corpuscles, stimulates arteries and sluggish menstrual discharge, and also the autonomic nervous system. Imbalances can show themselves in illnesses, such as piles, sciatica, prostate problems, depleted vitality, anaemia, sluggish menstrual discharge, total depletion and hopelessness, and lack of enthusiasm for life.

Base chakra

Colour	Organs and Endocrine Gland	Element	Sense	
Location	Parts of Body Affected	Planet	Emotion	Illness
Red	Kidneys; Bladder; Adrenals; Ovaries	Earth	Smell	Piles; Prostate; Sluggish
Coccyx	(especially) Testes	Saturn	Energy; Vitality;	menstrual discharge;
			Desire to live	Anaemia;
	Spine; Nervous system; Legs; Feet; Bones; Large intestine			Depleted vitality; Total depletion and hopelessness; Sciatica

The second or sacral chakra

The sacral chakra lies at the bottom of the sacrum or, when seen at the front, from the top of the pubic bone to just under the belly button, and is often seen as a wheel of red-orange light. It controls the genito-urinary system and is related to sexual activity and the reproductive organs. It is our creative area.

This chakra draws in energy from the earth's magnetic field through the feet. This energy is distributed and absorbed by all parts of the body. The chakra is associated with breathing, which increases absorption of these 'light photon particles'. Therefore, it influences the skin, lungs, and the immune and lymphatic system.

The second chakra influences the emotional levels of energy, as does the third chakra. It is associated with warm, positive stimulating vital processes of assimilation and absorption. When depleted it produces such emotions as anxiety and fear.

The orange ray of this chakra increases oxygen – breathing down to the belly will help the lungs, menstrual cramps, and reproductive problems. The orange ray releases gas, draws boils and brings abscesses to a head. It energises the immune system and stimulates the mother's milk production after she has given birth. It can have a calming effect on the adrenals, and also nourishes the kidneys.

Sacral chakra

Colour	Organs and Endocrine Gland	Element	Sense	
Location	Parts of Body Affected	Planet	Emotion	Illness
Orange-red	Kidneys; Bladder; Adrenals (especially);	Water	Taste	Diabetes; Cancer;
Bottom of sacrum and at front halfway between pubis/navel	Ovaries; Gonads (prostate) Skin; Lungs; Lymphatic system; Immune system	Jupiter	Fear; Anxiety	Menstrual cramps and reproductive problems; Premature ejaculation; Inability to to achieve erection and (in women) no orgasm; Poor urinary control or other urinary problems

The third or stomach chakra

The third chakra is located in the stomach area, above the navel. It can be seen as a wheel of yellow-green light. This chakra is closely linked to the parasympathetic nervous system. It can be a weak area for some people, an area where someone can easily feel hit by strong emotions, or have stomach problems from excess acidity or ulcers. It is the area where people fold their arms across their stomachs when they feel threatened by someone else. This centre is strongly connected to the emotions and to the emotional state.

This chakra controls the digestion and absorption of nutrients into the system, i.e. the stomach, diaphragm, duodenum, gall-bladder, liver, spleen and pancreas.

Working on this chakra can be helpful in cases of depression and anxiety; it helps intellectual debility and reinforces self-confidence and courage.

It stimulates the lymphatic glands, liver, gall-bladder, eyes, ears and also helps the elimination of excess calcium. It helps to loosen deposits of lime which cause arthritis; it loosens congestion and mucus in various parts of the body. This chakra is like the organising brain of the nervous system.

Growth and opening of this centre is impeded by misuse of power, domination, aggressive behaviour, guilt, doubt, indulging in depression, overeating or any form of over-consumption, and fear.

Stomach or solar plexus chakra

Colour	Organs and Endocrine Gland	Element	Sense	
Location	Parts of Body Affected	Planet	Emotion	Illness
Yellow-green	Pancreas; Andrenals; Stomach; Duodenum;	Fire	Sight	Ulcers; Cancer; Poor digestion;
Above navel	Liver; Gall-bladder; Diaphragm	Mars	Courage; Self-confidence	Depression; Lethargy; Rapid mood swings; Mental illness; Lack of confidence and courage

The fourth or heart chakra

The heart chakra is situated at the front, midway between the breasts, or, when seen at the back, between the shoulder-blades. It is sometimes seen as a wheel of golden or red light. It is the first of the higher level chakras.

This chakra controls the heart and the circulation of blood; it controls the vagus nerve, the largest nerve in the parasympathetic nervous system. It also controls the arms and the hands.

When this centre is well-balanced and open, you will experience compassion and great caring, and a sense of oneness with others. It is here that you develop a constant attitude of optimism, no matter what kind of difficulties you encounter; it is here that you continue to feel confident and optimistic that situations in life will improve.

As the heart chakra also controls the arms and the hands, your sense of touch will become more refined and subtle as this centre opens.

Working on this chakra helps to decongest the body, dissolve blood clots and heal infections. Always proceed with the greatest care when working in this area.

Negative aspects of this chakra involve oversentimentality, envy, jealousy, hard-heartedness, storing up possessions in order to feel safe, and holding materialistic values. Illnesses that can occur when this chakra is out of balance are heart and circulatory problems, angina, stroke, arthritis, epileptic fits. Personality disorders associated with this chakra include schizophrenia, paranoia, avarice, selfishness.

The heart energy may be damaged by pressure of work, overeating, drinking, smoking, drugs, body posture, and any form of physical or emotional holding on.

Heart chakra

Colour	Organs and Endocrine Gland	Element	Sense	
Location	Parts of Body Affected	Planet	Emotion	Illness
Gold-red	Thymus	Air	Touch	Heart attack; Stroke; Angina;
Heart	Heart	Venus	Unconditional love; Joy; Aliveness; Forgiveness; Feeling oneness with all living things; Harmony; Affinity with nature	Blood pressure; Epileptic fits; Arthritis; Schizophrenia; Paranoia; Avarice (extreme) Selfishness; Insecurity; Storing up of possessions to feel safe; Envy; Jealousy; Hatred

The fifth or throat chakra

The next chakra is the fifth, or throat chakra, which is situated at the throat, where it can be seen as a wheel of blue-violet light. This chakra controls the respiratory system, the vocal cords, the thyroid and the parathyroids, the pharyngeal and laryngeal nerve plexuses and the ears.

This is our centre for self-expression, devotion, idealism, commitment, strength of purpose and, therefore, patience and endurance. It is the centre for authoritative, balanced and compassionate use of power, especially the power of the voice, words and language. The throat centre is the centre through which we talk, sing and communicate with others. It can affect the glandular structure throughout the body. Whenever we use this centre in a negative way, for example when we use venomous words, the throat chakra will shut down and this can affect the thyroid, parathyroids, or the vocal cords. Imbalances can cause asthma, allergies, laryngitis, sore throat or problems in communication.

Negative expressions of this chakra are energy loss through excessive talking or idle chatter, 'bad mouthing' situations or people, the power of hypnotic dependence, destructive effects of dissonant and discordant sound, music, machinery, etc., smoking, shallow breathing, neck and throat tension, smugness, self-satisfaction, being dogmatic, melancholia, fanaticism, continuously seeking authority or being too authoritarian, rigidity, being ultra-conservative.

Illnesses that relate to this chakra are tonsillitis, laryngitis, throat cancer, swollen glands, sore throat, asthma, allergies.

Throat chakra

Colour	Organs and Endocrine Gland	Element	Sense	
Location	Parts of Body Affected	Planet	Emotion	Illness
Blue-violet	Thyroid; Parathyroids	Ether	Hearing	Thyroid problems; Flu;
Throat	Nervous system; Lungs; Vocal cords; Ears	Mercury	Self-expression; Devotion; Commit-ment; Compassion-ate use of power, especially power of voice; Words; Language	Swollen glands; Sore throat; Tonsillitis; Laryngitis; Throat cancer; Asthma; Allergies; Melancholia; Fanaticism; Rigidity; Neck and throat tension

The sixth or brow chakra

The brow chakra is located at the area between the eyebrows. To find its exact location, draw a line from the top of one ear across the forehead to the top of the other ear; then draw a line over the midline of the head down towards the tip of the nose; where the two lines cross is the area where the brow chakra, also called third eye or spiritual eye, is found. It is seen as a white light and controls the pineal gland and the pituitary gland. When awakening the chakras, begin by activating the brow chakra first. When awakened, it has the ability to release old habit patterns and can then help to awaken the lower chakras safely.

Once this chakra is developed and awakened it will give great mental clarity and insight. Coming from a source of deep knowledge and wisdom, it confers the ability to remain calm, whatever the circumstances. By working on this chakra it is possible to increase perception, abstract thought, intellect and awareness, and to develop a heightened sensitivity.

Exercise

The following exercise can be useful when developing the brow chakra and will help to quieten and calm the mind. Sit on the floor with the legs crossed and the spine straight. Breathe in slowly and deeply; continue to do this for a couple of minutes. Touch the forehead at the point of the spiritual eye for a couple of minutes. Then, bring the hand down and allow the gaze to float up towards the point you were touching on the forehead, as if you were following a lark into the heavens. Keep the head still, concentrate on the point on the forehead, and enjoy the feeling of lightness and joy that the lark brings.

Brow chakra or third/spiritual eye

Colour	Organs and Endocrine Gland	Element	Sense	
Location	Parts of Body Affected	Planet	Emotion	Illness
White	Pineal; Pituitary glands; Brain	Sun and moon	Heightened sensitivity and awareness; Abstract thought; Intuition; Inspiration	Schizophrenia; other mental illness; Negative thought forms
Forehead				

The seventh chakra or crown chakra

The crown chakra is located at the top of the head and can be seen as a golden light. This chakra controls body and mind; it controls the pineal gland. When this chakra is fully awakened it will bring one to a state of pure consciousness, of self-realisation, where one goes beyond all feelings, emotions and desires, all activities of the mind. It is through this chakra that one can reach the highest possible state of consciousness.

Crown chakra

Colour	Organs and Endocrine Gland	Element	Sense	
Location	Parts of Body Affected	Planet	Emotion	Illness
Gold	Pineal gland		A state of bliss	
At top of head	Whole body			

In conclusion

There are different opinions about the position and the colours of the chakras. Some see the chakras on the front of the body, some on the back, slightly behind the spine, and some see them in quite different positions.

As far as colour is concerned, some people see a simple rainbow spectrum from red at the base to white light at the top. Others see the colours differently again. It is also thought that the colours change slightly, according to the health of the body, emotional moods and state of mind.

It is thought that the sacral chakra in each person is developed at the time of birth, and the stomach chakra towards adulthood. Further development, leading to the opening of the stomach chakra, is usually required. Many of us function through this chakra, which is closely related to emotions. The negative emotions of this chakra are fear, often coming from feeling threatened and, therefore insecurity, guilt, doubt, depression, domination, aggressive behaviour, anger, vanity, competition with others and misuse of power. These negative qualities impede growth and opening of this chakra. Quite often, a person has to go through much suffering and pain before he realises that he needs to let go of such a negative pattern.

Further development of the chakras usually happens naturally, as the causal or emotional body evolves. The emotional body is the place where we work out our emotions and where we store the wisdom we obtain from all our experiences.

It is possible to help development of the chakras and to raise one's state of consciousness by way of meditation. Consciousness consists of self-awareness: being aware of oneself, one's thoughts, actions, feelings, and spiritual will, which follows self-awareness. The spiritual will brings the urge to establish harmony and sensitivity in dealing with others.

A note on safety

Much care and guidance is needed when working on the chakras. Premature opening of the chakras can lead to all sorts of aural and visual disturbances, and a range of effects from nervous tension to obsession.

Premature opening of the stomach chakra is especially dangerous. As mentioned before, development of the brow chakra before development of the other chakras is the suggested course of action. It is considered quite safe to exercise and meditate on this chakra.

Some warning needs to be given on prolonged concentration on the lower chakras, as this can cause a change in the activities of the associated endocrine glands. This could create imbalances in the body or its nervous and glandular system.

Shen Tao acupressure will automatically help to rebalance the chakras, and in a developed form works on the subtle levels of the physical body. In addition to Shen Tao, we can also treat ourselves by visualising very strongly the clear colour of each chakra, like sunlight through stained glass, seeing the whole area of the chakra and the body richly filled with glowing colour. If a chakra area feels in need of healing it is helpful to do this visualisation twice a day for five minutes in a quiet, peaceful place. When healing the chakras and chakra area it is important to take care of the physical energy balance as well by avoiding damaging foodstuffs for the corresponding organs (see section on food in Chapter 3).

Re-energising exercise

Sit comfortably. Relax as completely as possible. Concentrate on your whole body; exhale and inhale deeply. After three minutes of deep breathing, allow the attention to travel up your body, from your toes to your navel. Then visualise a large white–blue ball of light inside and outside the whole of the abdominal region. Focus your energy on your abdomen for three minutes. Then, without losing the image of the white–blue light, create a smaller ball of white–pink light and place this ball of light in position at the heart centre. Focus your energy there and breathe for three minutes.

Next, move up to the head and create a ball of white–golden light around your head and neck, whilst still visualising the white–blue light around your abdomen and the white–pink light around your heart centre. Focus your energy on your head and try to visualise each part of your head for another three minutes.

Finally, visualise your whole body within a white energy field in the shape of a luminous egg, and repeat the following affirmation silently: 'May peace and harmony reign within my whole being'. Gently and quietly bring your attention back into the room, keep breathing for another three minutes and then open your eyes.

This exercise is best done in the morning, before you start the day. It helps to cleanse and purify the body and to bring harmony to both mind and spirit.

5

SELF-TREATMENT: SINGLE POINT FIRST AID – QUICK REFERENCE

As acupressure needs no special equipment and can be practised easily at any time and in any place, it is particularly useful for self-treatment, either as first aid for a particular problem or as a more general means for relieving stress or restoring vitality.

Single point stress and pain relief points can be massaged or held at any time for about a minute. Finding the correct location of the points is important and the various illustrations in this book will give you quite a clear idea of how to do this. When you have studied the illustration concerned, you may find that your hands will intuitively lead you to the points. But if this does not come naturally, then you may notice that the skin where the point is located feels slightly different. For example, it could be a bit harder or tighter or lumpier, or it could be slightly softer, or there could be a slight dip in the skin, or it might feel slightly electric or numb or warmer or cooler, or you could find that that particular point feels quite painful or tender in some way. As your fingers become more sensitive you can feel these differences through clothing as well as on the bare skin.

If you place the fingertip of your middle finger on the right spot, you may sense a slight pulsation, which is different from that on the skin surrounding the point. To start with, it is a good idea to focus with your eyes closed, and as you become more familiar with the feel of the points, accurate location of them will become much easier.

If you are rebalancing a current condition, find a quiet place where you will not be disturbed. First, take your pulse reading (see page 88) and make a note of which meridians are full or empty, fast or slow. You will soon know what is normal, or balanced, for you. Make a choice of which points you are going to use from the repertoire (see page 105). Begin by relaxing as much as possible (sometimes your own bed is the best place to work), and breathing in 'Light and Healing Energy' (as described on pages 7–8), which flows to your heart, then down your arms to your fingertips. Wherever possible, make an energy circuit by holding the same point on each side, using both hands. Do not work for more than one hour. You can activate the points in different ways, according to what you find is best for you.

Movement

Spiral your fingertips clockwise to draw energy to a point that feels weak or depleted. Spiral anticlockwise to disperse a feeling of blockage, tension or pain. Gentle tapping also draws energy to the point. Placing the centre of your palm on a point will bring a lot of warmth and healing energy.

Depth of pressure

You can touch lightly sending the energy through your fingertips, or gradually press deeply until you contact the area of pain which will gradually ease. Find out which method works for you.

Length of holding

If you feel a pulsing developing under your fingertips, hold your fingers still for 30 seconds. This means you have called the qi to the point. For tense or painful areas you can hold the point for up to five minutes.

Self-treatment, using single points, step-by-step

The method to use for the points on the following diagrams is to press firmly for 1 to 2 minutes and massage clockwise if wished. Self-treatment is most effective if done daily, morning and evening, until symptoms ease.

Some safety considerations for self-treatment

- If you only need to use one or two points, make the habit of activating them early morning and when going to bed.

- Do not treat yourself just before a large meal and wait for one hour after eating a meal.

- Be careful not to over-treat, especially any abdominal points. Remember *more is not necessarily better.*

- Do not treat the abdomen when pregnant.

- Never press any point suddenly or with too intense pressure, and be aware of sensitive places on the body.

- Do not work near burns or areas of infection, or over new scars.

- It is important to rest and keep warm after treating yourself for any length of time.

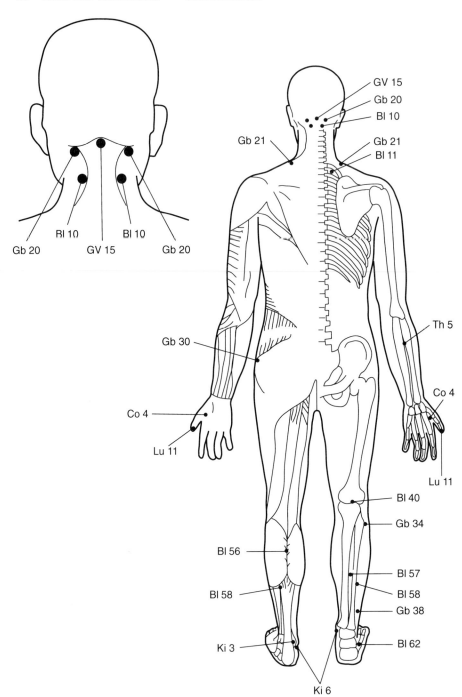

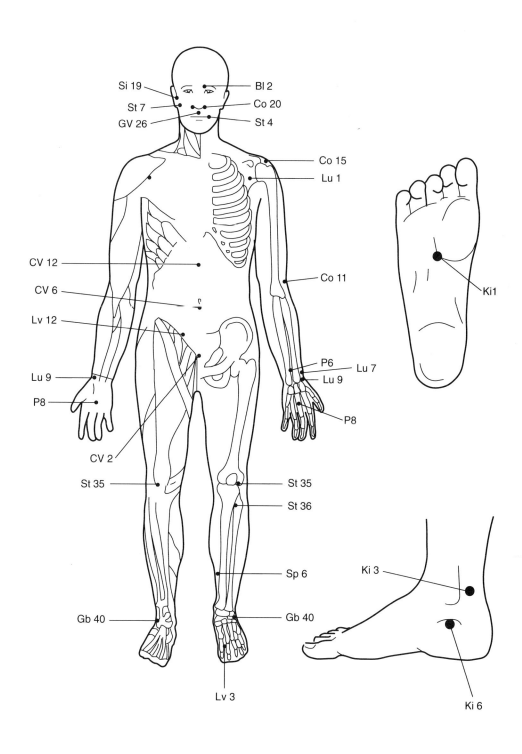

Arthritis

There are many different kinds of arthritis, including osteoarthritis and rheumatoid arthritis. However, for self-treatment, the acupoints given here will be generally helpful.

Arthritis often affects people who have experienced grief, anger, frustration and even hatred, and who may have suppressed these feelings. It can also affect people who have been unable to express their creativity. Subtle relief can often be experienced from these emotions by taking some of the flower remedies. Bach's Rescue Remedy is particularly helpful during periods of stress.

Professional help

Visit your GP or complementary practitioner of your choice for an initial diagnosis. In addition, it would be helpful to have dietary advice from a nutrition therapist. Homoeopathic treatment often gives good results.

Dietary advice

It is essential to make dietary changes, as unsuitable foods may well have been a contributory factor in the condition. Reduce acid-forming foods, animal fats and red meat. Avoid tea, coffee, alcohol, salt, spices, sugar, cheese, excess bread, grains or citrus fruits and drinks. Rely heavily on fruit and vegetables to cleanse the system; one day a week eating only fruit and fruit juice is beneficial (but *not* bananas). The following vitamins and minerals may help: vitamins E, B, C; niacinamids, calcium and magnesium. For some people Devil's Claw, and anti-inflammatory extract of lipid mussel (herbal preparations) may be helpful.

Other recommendations

- Take gentle regular exercise; yoga with a good teacher is beneficial.

- Treat the affected part with aromatherapy oils and use gentle massage. Heat treatment before application of the oils can sometimes help, although some swellings respond better to ice-packs. *Note:* it is important to move the affected joint as much as possible, immediately after massage, otherwise the heat can cause congestion and this will make the condition worse rather than better.

- Improve elimination of toxins, for example by dry skin brushing or taking mineral or seaweed baths.

Arthritis of the neck

Professional help

See the general advice given for arthritis, above.

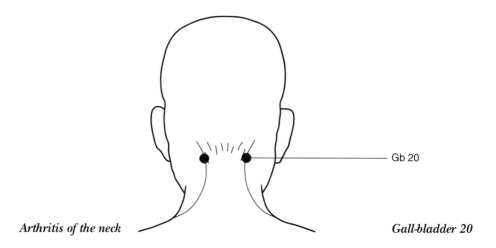

Arthritis of the neck   *Gall-bladder 20*

Dietary advice

See the dietary advice given for arthritis, above.

Other recommendations

- Gentle, regular exercise is beneficial, for example neck stretching and rolling the head from side to side, backwards and forwards and going around in a circle, starting from the right side rolling forwards, up to the left, and then backwards.

- Yoga is also very helpful.

- Treat the affected part with aromatherapy oils and use gentle massage. Some of the oils that can be used are eucalyptus, lemon, thyme, chamomile, juniper, marjoram, rosemary, ginger, benzoin or sandalwood. You can make up a mixture of 2 or 3 oils in 1 dessertspoonful of almond or grapeseed oil, using 2 or 3 drops of each of your chosen oils. Try, for example, one of the following mixtures: to 1 dessertspoon almond or grapeseed oil add: 3 drops ginger, 3 drops rosemary, 3 drops lemon; or 1 drop benzoin, 3 drops marjoram, 4 drops lemon; or 2 drops sandalwood, 3 drops lemon, 2 drops ginger; or 2 drops German chamomile, 3 drops eucalyptus, 3 drops marjoram.

- Heat-treatment before application of the oils can sometimes help, but some swellings respond better to ice-packs.

Acupressure points

Gall-bladder 20   This point lies in the hollow at the base of the skull, on each side of the spine, where the hairline starts. Activate both sides using the middle fingers of each hand to press in and up under the skull.

Arthritis of the shoulder

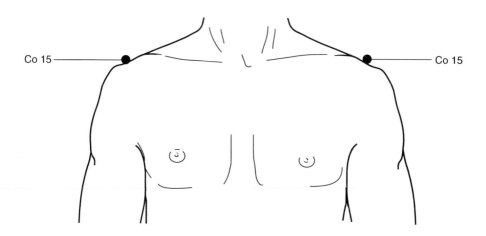

Co 15 ———————————————————— Co 15

Arthritis of the shoulders

Colon (15)

Professional help

See the general advice given for arthritis, on page 42.

Dietary advice

See the dietary advice given for arthritis, on page 42.

Other recommendations

- Gentle exercise to keep the area mobile will help, for example, loosening and rolling the shoulders backwards and forwards.
- Yoga is helpful.
- Treat the affected part with aromatherapy oils and use gentle massage. Suitable oils and suggestions for mixtures are given on page 43, under arthritis of the neck.
- Heat treatment before appliction of the oils can sometimes help, but some swellings respond better to ice-packs.

Acupressure points

Colon 15   This point is found in the depression between the top of the arm and the collarbone, at the top of the shoulder, towards the front. Press in and towards the top of the arm.

Arthritis of the elbow

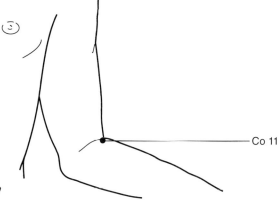

Arthritis of the elbow — Co 11 — *Colon 11*

Professional help

See the general advice given for arthritis, on page 42.

Dietary advice

See the dietary advice given for arthritis, on page 42.

Other recommendations

- Gentle exercise to keep the area mobile will help, for example, loosening and rolling the arms backwards and forwards.

- Yoga is also helpful.

- Treat the affected part with aromatherapy oils and use gentle massage. Some of the oils that can be used are frankincense, lemon, thyme, chamomile, juniper, marjoram, rosemary, ginger, benzoin, sandalwood, peppermint. You can make up a mixture of 2 or 3 oils in 1 dessertspoonful of almond or grapeseed oil, using 2 or 3 drops of your chosen oils. Try for example one of the following mixtures: to 1 dessertspoonful almond oil or grapeseed oil add: 2 drops frankincense, 3 drops lavender, 3 drops lemon; or 3 drops thyme, 3 drops lemon, 3 drops lavender; or 2 drops sandalwood, 3 drops lemon, 2 drops ginger; or 2 drops German chamomile, 3 drops juniper berry, 3 drops marjoram.

- Heat-treatment before application of the oils can sometimes help, but some swellings respond better to ice-packs.

Acupressure points

Colon 11   This point is found at the end of the elbow crease, with the arm bent; press down towards the funny bone.

Arthritis of the wrist

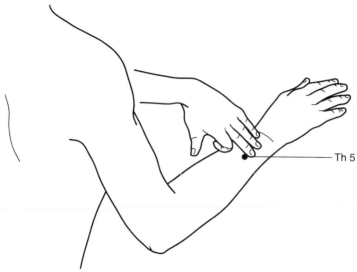

Th 5

Arthritis of the wrist   *Triple heater 5*

Professional help

See the general advice given for arthritis, on page 42.

Dietary advice

See the dietary advice given for arthritis, on page 42.

Other recommendations

- Gentle exercise to keep the area mobile will help, for example flexing and rolling the wrists.

- Yoga is also helpful.

- Treat the affected part with aromatherapy oils and use gentle massage. See the suggestions for oils and mixtures, given for arthritis of the elbow, on page 45.

- Heat-treatment before application of the oils can sometimes help, but some swellings respond better to ice-packs.

Acupressure points

Triple Heater 5   This point lies 3 finger widths above the wrist crease, on the back of the hand and centrally in line with the middle finger. Press inwards, towards the centre of the wrist.

Arthritis of the hand

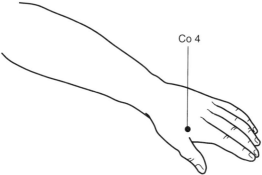

Co 4

Arthritis of the hand   *Colon 4*

Professional help

See the general advice given for arthritis, on page 42.

Dietary advice

See the dietary advice given for arthritis, on page 42.

Other recommendations

- Gentle exercise is beneficial, for example flexing and stretching the hands and fingers, or, gently pulling the fingers and rotating the fingers whilst holding them at the tip with the other hand.

- Yoga is also helpful.

- Treat the affected part with aromatherapy oils and use gentle massage. Some of the oils that can be used are frankincense, lemon, chamomile, juniper, marjoram, ginger, sandalwood, lavender, peppermint. You can make up a mixture of 2 or 3 oils in 1 dessertspoonful of almond or grapeseed oil, using 2 or 3 drops of each of your chosen oils. Try for example one of the following mixtures: to 1 dessertspoonful almond oil or grapeseed oil add: 2 drops benzoin, 4 drops lavender, 3 drops lemon; or 2 drops peppermint, 3 drops lavender, 2 drops frankincense.

- Heat-treatment before application of the oils can sometimes help, but some swellings respond better to ice-packs.

Acupressure points

Colon 4   This point is a major elimination point and is found at the end of the crease when a fist is made, in the web between the thumb and finger. Press towards the fingerbone of the hand.

Arthritis of the hip

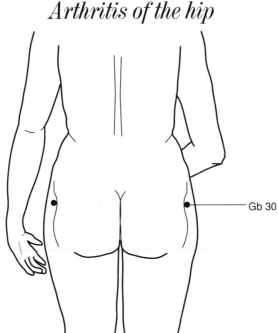

Arthritis of the hip   *Gall-bladder 30*

Professional help

See the general advice given for arthritis, on page 42.

Dietary advice

See the dietary advice given for arthritis, on page 42.

Other recommendations

- With this condition it is important not to put on weight. If you are overweight, eat fewer carbohydrates and fats and cut down on sugar.

- For additional self-treatment take gentle exercise.

- Yoga is particularly beneficial.

- Treat the affected part with aromatherapy oils and use gentle massage. Some of the oils that can be used are frankincense, lemon, chamomile, juniper, marjoram, ginger, sandalwood, lavender, eucalyptus and black pepper. You can make up a mixture of 2 or 3 oils in 1 dessertspoonful of almond or grapeseed oil, using 2 or 3 drops of each of your chosen oils. Try one of the following mixtures: to 1 dessertspoonful almond oil or grapeseed oil add: 3 drops rosemary, 2 drops ginger, 3 drops lavender; or 3 drops lavender, 3 drops marjoram, 3 drops lemon; or 2 drops sandalwood, 2 drops ginger, 3 drops Roman chamomile; or 2 drops black pepper, 3 drops lemon, 3 drops juniper berry.

- Application of heat-treatment before you massage with the oils, such as infrared light, may help.

- Hot baths or hot compresses can also help, but some swellings respond better to ice-packs.

Acupressure points

Gall-bladder 30   This point is found in the hollow at the side of the hips at the joint between the pelvis and leg. Press strongly inwards.

Arthritis of the knee

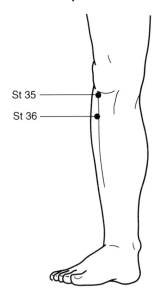

St 35

St 36

Arthritis of the knee   *Stomach 35-36*

Professional help
See the general advice given for arthritis, on page 42.

Dietary advice
See the dietary advice given for arthritis, on page 42.

Other recommendations

- With this condition it is important not to put on weight. If you are overweight, cut down on carbohydrates and fats.

- For additional self-treatment take gentle exercise.

- Yoga can be very beneficial.
- Treat the affected part with aromatherapy oils and use gentle massage. See the suggestions for oils and mixtures of oils on page 48, under arthritis of the hip.
- Application of heat-treatment before you massage with the oils, such as infrared light, may help.
- Hot baths or hot compresses can be helpful, but some swellings respond better to ice-packs.

Acupressure points

Stomach 36   This is a very important point for arthritis. It is found 3 thumb widths under the kneecap, in the hollow on the *outer edge* of the shin. Press firmly inwards.

Stomach 35   This point is just *under* the kneecap in the *depression on the outer edge* of the leg. Press in under the kneecap.

Arthritis of the ankle

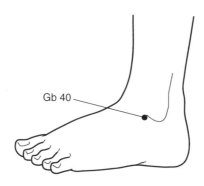

Gb 40

Arthritis of the ankle   *Gall-bladder 40*

Professional help

See the general advice for arthritis, on page 42.

Dietary advice

See the dietary advice for arthritis, on page 42.

Other recommendations

- With this condition, it is important not to put on weight. If you are overweight, cut down on your carbohydrates and fats.
- For additional self-treatment, take gentle exercise.
- Yoga can be very beneficial.

- Gentle exercise to keep the area mobile will help, such as loosening and circling the ankles.

- Treat the affected part with aromatherapy oils and use gentle massage. Some of the oils that can be used are eucalyptus, lemon, thyme, chamomile, juniper, marjoram, rosemary, ginger, benzoin, sandalwood, peppermint. You can make up a mixture of 2 or 3 oils in 1 dessertspoonful of almond or grapeseed oil, using 2 or 3 drops of each of your chosen oils. Try for example one of the following mixtures: to 1 dessertspoonful almond oil or grapeseed oil add: 2 drops rosemary, 3 drops lavender, 3 drops lemon; or 3 drops juniper, 3 drops marjoram, 2 drops sandalwood; or 2 drops sandalwood, 3 drops lemon, 2 drops ginger; or 2 drops black pepper, 3 drops lemon, 3 drops juniper berry.

- Application of heat-treatment before you massage with the oils, such as infrared light, may help.

- Hot baths or hot compresses can be helpful, but some swellings respond better to ice-packs.

Acupressure points

Gall-bladder 40   This point is found in the depression under the outer ankle bone, towards the top of the foot. Press towards the centre of the foot.

Catarrh

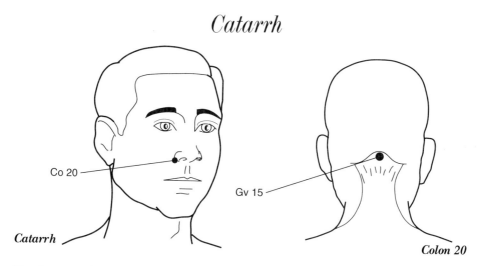

Co 20

Gv 15

Catarrh

Colon 20

Professional help

If chronic, consult your GP, homoeopath or other complementary practitioner of your choice. Diet may be a contributary factor, so visit a nutrition therapist. It may be helpful to try herbal or homoeopathic medicine from your local chemist or healthfood shop.

Dietary advice

Avoid mucus-forming dairy products, eggs and too many bananas; avoid fried foods, sweets, junk foods, sugar, excess carbohydrates. Increase the intake of cleansing foods (fruit and fresh green vegetables). Drink plenty of water.

Other recommendations

- Steam inhalations are very beneficial. Fill a bowl with boiling water, add some essential oils (for example 2 drops peppermint, 1 drop rosemary, 1 drop lavender), mix well. Keep your head under a towel, above the bowl and inhale for approximately 10 minutes.

- In the evening, rub your chest and back with a mixture of aromatherapy oils. Use grapeseed or almond oil as a base and add essential oils, such as rosemary, eucalyptus, lavender or sandalwood. Use 2 or 3 oils together and never more than 2–3 drops of each.

- Catarrh may be helped by improving elimination. It is important to avoid constipation. Do daily dry skin brushing to improve elimination from the skin also.

- Colonic irrigation is sometimes appropriate for this condition.

- Increase outdoor exercise. Swimming is excellent for general health and improving the circulation.

Acupressure points

Governing Vessel 15   Find this point at the back of the head, centrally under the base of the skull at the top of the spine. Press under the skull and up.

Colon 20   This point is found on each side of the nose, close to the base of the nostrils on the cheek. Press each side with the fingers of both hands.

Claustrophobia

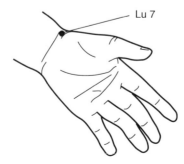

Lu 7

Claustrophobia   *Lung 7*

Professional help

Consult your GP or complementary practitioner. Counselling or psychotherapy may be appropriate.

Dietary advice

A nutrition therapist could help to cleanse the system. In Chinese medicine, claustrophobia has a connection with the metal element lung/colon. Therefore, a diet low in fats and dairy products would be helpful in removing the stress from these meridians.

Other recommendations

- Professionally prescribed flower remedies can be very effective (see your nearest therapist for an assessment).

- Meditation and deep relaxation exercises can be beneficial, as can yoga, for restoring inner calm.

Acupressure points

Lung 9   This is found on the inner wrist crease, under the base of the thumb. Press firmly inwards.

Colds

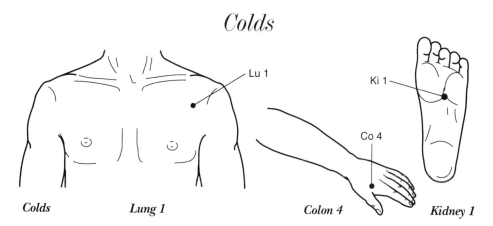

| Colds | Lung 1 | Colon 4 | Kidney 1 |

Professional help

Consult your GP or complementary practitioner if chronic.

Dietary advice

A nutrition therapist could help to cleanse the system. It is better to avoid aspirin and other preparations which only suppress the infection. A cold is a natural toxic elimination process. Drink plenty of water, preferably mineral water to help detoxification.

Other recommendations

- Try to get plenty of rest.

Acupressure points

Colon 4   This point is a major elimination point and is found at the end of the crease when a fist is made, in the web between the thumb and finger. Press towards the fingerbone on the hand.

Lung 1   This point is 2 fingers width down from the collarbone on the outer edge of the ribcage. Press in and against the ribs.

Kidney 1   This point is found on the soles of the feet, centrally, just behind the padded ball of the foot. Press inwards (*note:* this point is sometimes sensitive, so increase the pressure gently).

Colitis

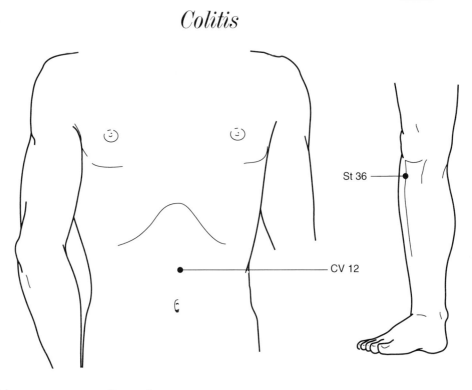

Colitis   *Conception Vessel 12*   *Stomach 36*

Professional help

Consult your GP or complementary practitioner for an initial diagnosis. Dietary factors may be involved, so visit a nutrition therapist. Try herbal medicine and/or homoeopathy.

Dietary advice

Roughage does *not* cause colitis; a high-fibre diet is the best prevention and cure. However, in the acute stages, a bland low-fibre diet is necessary. Slippery elm is very helpful as is brown rice. Gradually introduce steamed vegetables and stewed fruit. Follow a meat-free diet for several months and avoid all fried foods. The following vitamins and minerals may help: multi-vitamin and a B complex; calcium.

Other recommendations

- Colonic irrigation may be appropriate at the onset of the condition.
- Cold compresses over the abdomen may help.
- Meditation and deep relaxation will calm the nervous system.

Acupressure points

Conception Vessel 12   This point lies centrally, midway between the bottom of the breastbone and the navel. Press firmly inwards.
Stomach 36   This point is found 3 thumb widths under the kneecap, in the hollow on the *outer edge* of the shin. Press firmly inwards.

Cystitis

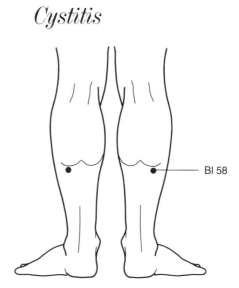

BI 58

Cystitis   *Bladder 58*

Professional help

Consult your GP or a complementary practitioner of your choice for a diagnosis and treatment. Visit a nutrition therapist, as diet is often a factor in this condition.

Dietary advice

There is usually a need for a detoxing diet: avoid alcohol, sugar and antibiotics. Drink plenty of water, fruit juices and herbal teas, at least 2 pints a day, but avoid tea and coffee. Include extra green vegetables and plenty of fruit. Vitamins and other remedies would be beneficial, such as a multi-vitamin complex. Try Goldenseal tea, 3 times a day; this is well-known for its healing properties.

Other recommendations

- As additional self-treatment apply aromatherapy. Make up a mixture of 1 dessertspoonful almond oil and 2 drops bergamot, 2 drops lavender and 1 drop chamomile essential oils and massage the lower abdomen, hips and lower back with this, until you experience relief from the symptoms – this can vary from a few days to a couple of weeks.

- If there is a lot of pain, use a hot compress with chamomile oil over the lower abdomen.

Acupressure points

Bladder 58   This point lies towards the back of the lower leg, on the outer side and on the lower slope of the calf muscle. Press in towards the centre of the leg and up.

Dizziness, fainting

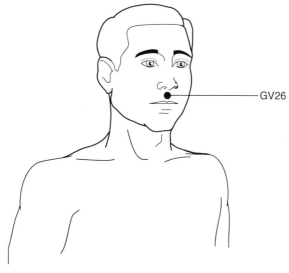

GV26

Dizziness, fainting

GV 26

Professional help

Consult your GP or a complementary practitioner of your choice. It may be helpful to visit a nutrition therapist and to try herbal or homoeopathic remedies.

Other recommendations

- Take as much rest as possible and keep warm. Have your blood pressure checked and get tested for anaemia.

- Meditation and relaxation may help if stress is the cause.

- Try back and neck massage, if possible with relaxing aromatherapy oils, such as German chamomile, rose and sandalwood.

- The cause may be related to liver problems from a Chinese medicine viewpoint. Therefore, if the problem is chronic, see a therapist for regular acupuncture or acupressure treatment.

Acupressure points

Governing Vessel 26   This point is found on the top of the lip, mid-way between the nose and the top lip. Press inwards.

Indigestion

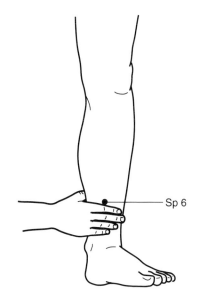

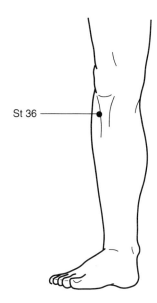

Indigestion

Spleen 6 and Stomach 36

Professional help

If this is long-term and severe, consult your GP or a complementary practitioner of your choice. Visit a nutrition therapist, as diet may be a significant factor in this condition. Try herbal medicine and/or homoeopathy.

Dietary advice

Indigestion could be related to a food imbalance or allergy. Too many raw, cold foods in winter may cause indigestion. Also an excess of dairy products causes digestive problems. Excess carbohydrates, coffee, tea and alcohol should be avoided, in addition to acid-forming foods. Overeating can aggravate this condition and drinking with meals should be avoided. Do not skip meals, eat too rapidly, or eat on the run. Do not eat a heavy meal late at night. Check for food allergies with a dietician.

Other recommendations

- Indigestion can be caused by emotional stress. Practise meditation and relaxation techniques to help relieve stress and tension.
- Try aromatherapy. Mix together 1 dessertspoonful almond oil with 3 drops mandarin and 3 drops fennel. Massage this over the stomach and solar plexus area.

Acupressure points

Spleen 6   This point is found 4 finger widths down from the crown of the inner ankle. Press against the bone.

Insomnia

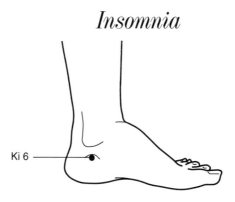

Ki 6

Insomnia   *Kidney 6*

Professional help

Consult your GP or complementary practitioner, if the problem is long-standing. If stress or personal problems are the cause, try psychotherapy or counselling.

Dietary advice

Do not eat heavy or rich food late at night, especially cheese and cream. Avoid coffee and excess alcohol. Some herbal remedies are available to help with insomnia, but try to avoid sleeping pills, unless absolutely necessary.

Other recommendations

- Before going to bed have a warm bath scented with aromatherapy oils, such as ylang ylang, rose, chamomile, neroli, petitgrain, geranium, juniper berry, marjoram or bergamot. Try one of the following mixtures: 2 drops rose, 2 drops bergamot, 2 drops geranium; or 2 drops ylang ylang, 2 drops bergamot, 2 drops geranium; or 1 drop neroli, 2 drops petitgrain and 2 drops bergamot; or 2 drops juniper berry, 2 drops marjoram and 2 drops geranium.

- Put a couple of drops of essential oil in a humidifier filled with water and hang it on the radiator in your bedroom.

- Alternatively, put a drop of essential oil on a tissue and keep that by your pillow.

- Some people find a hop pillow helpful.

Acupressure points

Kidney 6   This point lies directly under the inner ankle bone. Press in and up.
Bladder 62   This point lies directly under the outer ankle bone. Press in and up.

Joint problems

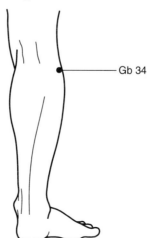

Gb 34

Joint problems   *Gall-bladder 34*

Professional help

Consult your GP or complementary practitioner of your choice. Visit a nutrition therapist. Try sound therapy, herbal medicine and/or homoeopathy.

Dietary advice

It is essential to make dietary changes, as unsuitable foods may well have been a contributory factor to the condition. Reduce acid-forming foods, animal fats and red meat. Avoid tea, coffee, alcohol, salt, spices, sugar, cheese, excess bread, grains or citrus fruits and drinks. Rely heavily on fruit and vegetables to cleanse the system. Try one day a week eating only fruit and fruit juice (but *not* bananas). The following vitamins and minerals may help: vitamins E, B, C; niacinamids, calcium and magnesium. For some people the herbal recommendations Devil's Claw and anti-inflammatory extract of lipid mussel may be useful.

Acupressure points

Gall-bladder 34   This point is found on the outer side of the knee, 4 finger widths down from the kneecap, in the hollow between the shin and the smaller leg bone. Press in and slightly up.

Kidney complaints

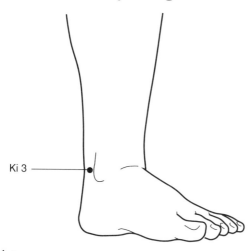

Kidney complaints   *Kidney 3*

Professional help

Consult your GP or complementary practitioner of your choice. Visit a nutrition therapist. Try herbal medicine and/or homoeopathy.

Dietary advice

With kidney complaints there is often the need for a detoxing diet and drinking more water. The condition may be due to a chill, or be aggravated by excess animal protein and milk. It can also be aggravated by an excess of antibiotics. The following vitamins and minerals may help: vitamin A and B complex, vitamin E; choline may also help to improve this condition. Parsley is very cleansing, eaten raw, in salads or made into a tea.

Other recommendations

- Keep the kidney area warm.

- Make sure you get plenty of rest.

- Geranium or lavender essential oils, either added to the bath or diluted with a carrier oil and used in an aromatherapy massage are soothing and cleansing.

Acupressure points

Kidney 3   This point is found in the hollow between the inner anklebone and the Achilles tendon. Press firmly inwards.

Laryngitis

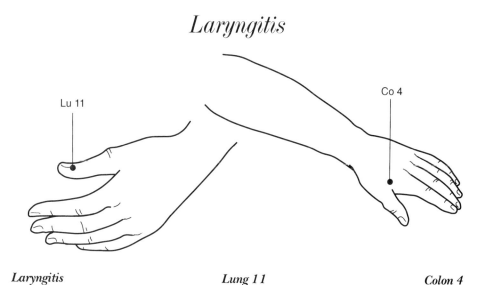

Lu 11

Co 4

Laryngitis   *Lung 11*   *Colon 4*

Professional help

Consult your GP or complementary practitioner of your choice. Visit a nutrition therapist. Try sound therapy, herbal medicine and/or homoeopathy.

Dietary advice

Try drinking hot water with lemon and honey, morning and evening. Go on to a cleansing diet, consisting mainly of fruit and vegetables while the condition is acute. The biochemic tissue salt calc phos (4 tablets every hour while acute) may prove beneficial.

Other recommendations

- Steam inhalations: fill up a bowl with boiling water and add 3 drops lavender and 2 drops sandalwood or benzoin. Mix well. Keep your head under a towel and above the bowl for 10 minutes.

- Avoid smoking or smoky or over-dry atmospheres.

- Rest the voice totally till the symptoms have subsided.

Acupressure points

Lung 11   This point is found at the bottom corner of the nail on the outer side of the thumb. Press vertically inwards.
Colon 4   This is a major elimination point. It lies at the end of the crease in the web between the finger and the thumb. Press towards the fingerbone on the hand.

Lumbago

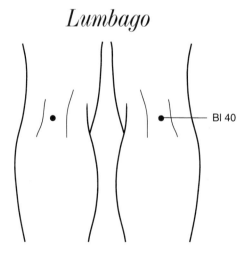

BI 40

Lumbago   *Bladder 40*

Professional help

Consult your GP or complementary practitioner of your choice. Try herbal medicine and/or homoeopathy. Regular treatments with an osteopath, cranio-sacral therapist and aromatherapist can be very beneficial. Always check with your doctor first for a slipped disc or a trapped nerve.

Dietary advice

Choose a light detoxing diet with plenty of fruit and vegetables and reduced dairy and wheat products. The following vitamins and minerals may also be helpful: vitamins B, C, E; calcium, magnesium.

Other recommendations

- Hot compresses, applied to the lower back, with aromatherapy oils as follows: fill a bowl with hot water, add 3 drops marjoram, 4 drops lavender and 3 drops ginger. Mix well. Soak a compress in the bowl and wring out slightly. Put over lower back and put a towel and a blanket over the compress. Meanwhile, keep the bowl containing the water warm. Replace the compress when cold. Repeat this 3 to 6 times. Do this at least 3 times a day, or as often as needed.

- Some people respond better to ice-cold compresses. If this is the case, rub the affected area with ice-cubes in circular movements, or put a bag of frozen peas on the lower back and leave for 5 minutes.

Acupressure points

Bladder 40   Centre of back of knee crease. Press inwards (*note:* this is not recommended if you suffer with varicose veins).

Migraine

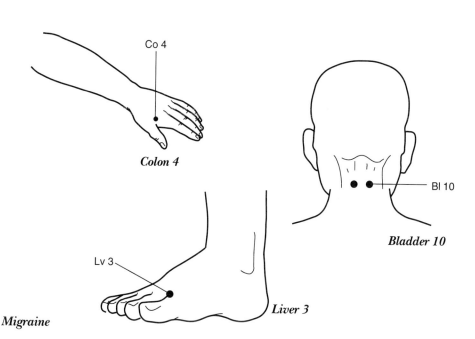

Co 4

Colon 4

Bl 10

Bladder 10

Lv 3

Liver 3

Migraine

Professional help

Consult your GP or complementary practitioner of your choice. If the problem is chronic, see a therapist for regular acupressure treatments, combined with aromatherapy or reflexology or cranio-sacral therapy.

Dietary advice

The diet usually needs complete revision. Avoid coffee, chocolate, dairy products (especially cheese) and alcohol. Increase the intake of green vegetables and fruit. A regular fast, eating fruit only for one day a week, may help. The following vitamins and other preparations may help: vitamin B complex; ferrum phos (4 tablets every $\frac{1}{2}$ hour whilst the condition is acute).

Other recommendations

- Avoid constipation and mental and emotional stress. Migraines can be the result of a driving personality. Insomnia can also be a causative factor.

- The combination of insufficient sleep, pressure of work and stress, together with the build up of too many liver-stressing foods, is often the trigger for a migraine attack. Rest, sleep and eat only fruit during, and for a while after, the attack.

- Have an ice-pack on the forehead simultaneously with a hot footbath.

- Sometimes the migraine is helped by taking an enema.

- A course of biochemic tissue salts can be good as a preventative.

- Cold compresses: fill a bowl with hot water and add 3 drops lavender oil and 1 drop peppermint oil. Mix well and let cool. Soak compress in bowl, wring out and place over forehead. Change as soon as compress is warm.

- Warm compresses: place warm compresses (use warm water with 3 drops marjoram) on the back of the neck, to increase the flow of blood to the head.

- Practise meditation and relaxation techniques.

Acupressure points

Colon 4   This is a major elimination point. It is found at the end of the crease in the web between the finger and the thumb. Press towards the fingerbone on the hand.

Bladder 10   This point is close to the sides of the spine at the top of the neck, under the skull. Activate both sides by pressing in and up.

Liver 3   This point lies in the web between the big toe and the next toe. Press in and up, towards the centre of the foot.

Motion sickness

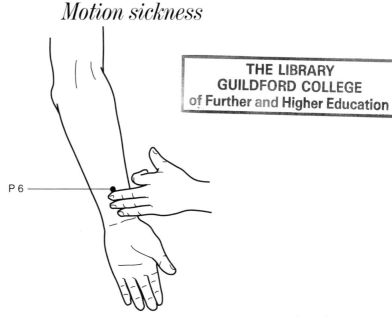

P 6

Motion sickness   *Pericardium (6)*

Professional help

Consult your GP or complementary practitioner of your choice. Try herbal medicine and/or homoeopathy.

Dietary advice

Avoid rich or heavy meals before or during travel. Drink plenty of water. There are some safe herbal remedies for motion sickness.

Other recommendations

- Avoid tight clothing or stuffy atmospheres.
- It may help to put a few drops of peppermint oil on a handkerchief to inhale.
- When flying, avoid reading too much. Rest the eyes and practise deep breathing.
- For car travel, it may be helpful to have a chain or cord in contact with the ground to provide some kind of 'earthing'.

Acupressure points

Pericardium 6   This point is found 3 finger widths above the wrist crease on the inner wrist, centrally on the line with the middle finger. Press towards the centre of the wrist.

Nausea and vomiting

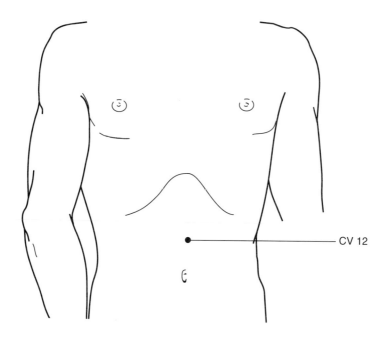

Nausea and vomiting   *Conception vessel 12*

Professional help

Consult your GP or a complementary practitioner if the problem is recurrent and if the cause is unknown.

Dietary advice

Drink fennel and peppermint tea regularly or fill a mug with hot water and the juice of half a lemon and some honey, and take this in the same way.

Other recommendations

- Mix 1 dessertspoonful almond oil with 2 drops bergamot and 3 drops fennel. Massage this into the abdomen and solar plexus area.

Acupressure points

Pericardium 6   This point is found 3 finger widths above the wrist crease on the line with the middle finger. Press towards the centre of the wrist.
Conception Vessel 12   This point lies centrally at the midpoint between the bottom of the breastbone and the navel. Press firmly inwards.

Neuralgia

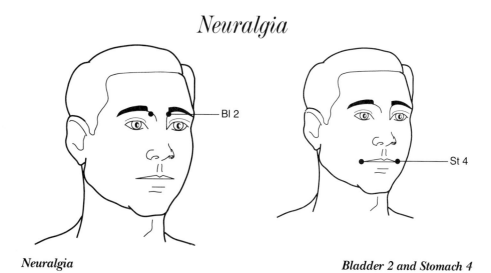

Neuralgia   ***Bladder 2 and Stomach 4***

Professional help

Consult your GP or complementary practitioner of your choice. Try herbal medicine and/or homoeopathy. It is important to see your doctor if the condition is persistent.

Dietary advice

Check for vitamin B deficiency. Brewer's yeast and kelp tablets or wheat germ oil will bring an improvement if there is a deficiency.

Other recommendations

- See an osteopath, chiropractor or cranio-sacral therapist to check the spine.
- Use cold compresses or rub with ice-cubes over the affected area or try alternate hot and cold compresses.
- Try winter-green oil as an external application, massaged in lightly.
- Massage the affected area gently to relieve the inflammation with an aromatherapy oil mixture of 1 dessertspoonful of almond oil and a few drops of German chamomile and marjoram.
- After massage apply the acupressure points.

Acupressure points

Bladder 2   This point is found at the inner end of the eyebrow. Press inwards.
Stomach 4   This point is close to the corners of the mouth. Press down towards the jaw.

Osteoarthritis

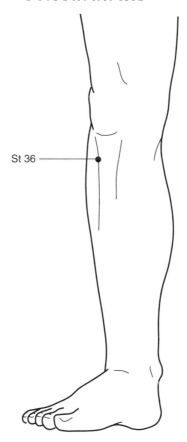

St 36

Osteoarthritis   *Stomach 36*

Professional help

Consult your GP or complementary practitioner of your choice. Try herbal medicine and/or homoeopathy. It will be helpful to combine acupressure with aromatherapy or homoeopathy.

Dietary advice

It is essential to make dietary changes, as unsuitable foods may well have been a contributory factor to the condition. Reduce acid-forming foods, animal fats and red meat. Avoid tea, coffee, alcohol, salt, spices, sugar, cheese, excess bread, grains and citrus fruits or drinks.

Acupressure points

Stomach 36   This is a major point for arthritis. It is found 3 thumb widths under the kneecap, in the hollow on the *outer edge* of the shin. Press inwards.

Pain

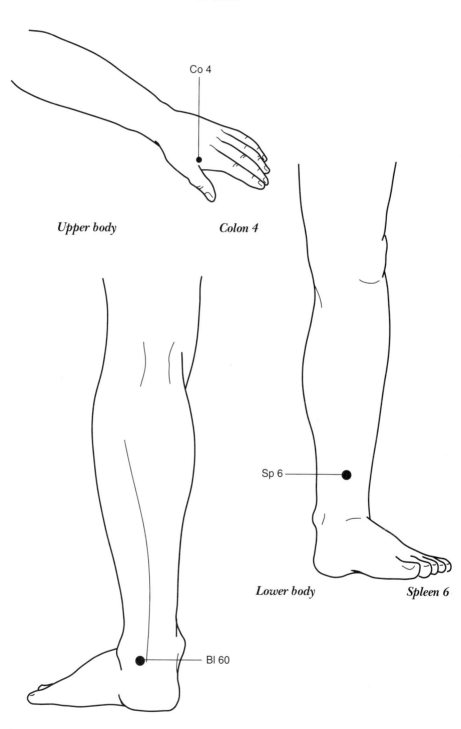

Upper body   **Colon 4**

Lower body   **Spleen 6**

Pain in general   **Bladder 60**

Professional help

Consult your GP or complementary practitioner of your choice. Pain is a warning signal from the body, so it is important to find its cause.

Dietary advice

Follow a detoxing diet as an initial step, while awaiting diagnosis of the pain from a professional medical practitioner.

Other recommendations

- Massage the affected area very gently with a mixture of 1 dessertspoonful almond oil and 3 drops lavender essential oil.

- Use flower remedies. If the pain is unexplained and cannot be cured, see a qualified therapist immediately.

Acupressure points

Bladder 60   This point is found in the hollow behind the outer ankle bone. Press in a little towards the ankle bone. Treat this point for general pain.

Colon 4   This point is a major elimination point. It lies at the end of the crease in the web between the finger and the thumb. Press towards the finger bone on the hand. Treat this point for pain in the upper body.

Spleen 6   This point lies 1 hand width above the crown of the inner ankle bone. Press inwards beside the bone. Treat this point for pain in the lower body.

Prolapse of the rectum (piles)

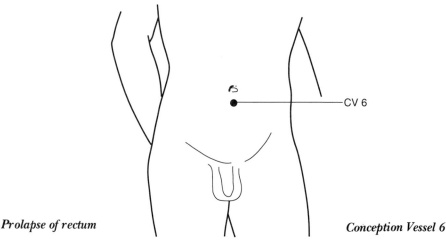

CV 6

Prolapse of rectum

Conception Vessel 6

Professional help

Consult your GP or complementary practitioner of your choice.

Dietary advice

Increase roughage and fibre to avoid constipation. Begin a cleansing diet, avoiding dairy products and foods which create acid. Take extra fruit and fresh green vegetables. Avoid tea, coffee and alcohol.

Other recommendations

- Lie down on the floor and pull up the muscles of the rectum; hold for 10 seconds; relax. Repeat this 8–10 times. Practise this in the morning or evening, at a time when convenient to you.

- After finishing the above exercise, press the acupoint and hold for 1–2 minutes.

Acupressure points

Conception Vessel 6   This point is found on the abdomen, 2 finger widths below the navel on the centre line. Press inwards firmly.

Prolapse of the uterus

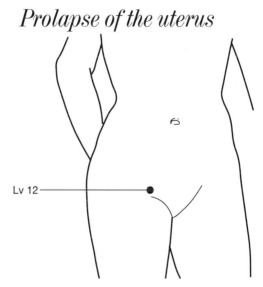

Lv 12

Prolapse of the uterus   *Liver 12*

Professional help

Consult your GP or complementary practitioner of your choice.

Dietary advice

A general cleansing diet with an increase in fruit and vegetables will tone the whole system.

Other recommendations

- The following exercise is helpful for the uterus. Lie down and pull up the uterus from the vagina. This should feel as if you need to urinate, but are stopping yourself by pulling in the muscles in that area. You can also do this exercise whilst standing, keeping your legs apart.

- Press the acupoint after the exercise and hold for 1–2 minutes.

Acupressure points

Liver 12   This point lies 2 finger widths above the pubic bone, and 1 hand width from the centre line. Press diagonally inwards.

Restless legs

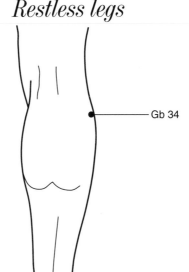

Gb 34

Restless legs   *Gall-bladder 34*

Professional help

Consult your GP or complementary practitioner of your choice. Try herbal medicine and/or homoeopathy.

Dietary advice

Avoid tea and coffee, as too much caffeine can cause this condition.

Other recommendations

- Massage the legs with a mixture of 1 dessertspoonful almond oil with 2 drops German chamomile oil.

Acupressure points

Gall-bladder 34   This point is found on the outer side of the knee, 4 finger widths down from the kneecap, in the hollow between the shin and the smaller leg bone. Press in and against the upper bone.

Ringing in the ears (Tinnitus)

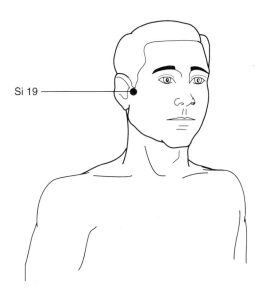

Si 19

Ringing in ears   *Small intestine 19*

Professional help

Consult your GP or complementary practitioner of your choice. Try herbal medicine and/or homoeopathy.

Dietary advice

Follow a detoxing diet and avoid tea and coffee.

Other recommendations

• Take extra rest and avoid stress.

Acupressure points

Small intestine 19   This point is found 1 finger width in front of the ear at the top of the cheekbone. Press inwards.

Sciatica in the leg

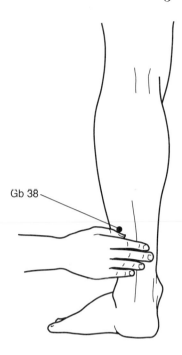

Sciatica in the leg   *Gall-bladder 38*

Professional help

Consult your GP or complementary practitioner of your choice. Try herbal medicine and/or homoeopathy. Reflexology, cranio-sacral therapy, painless spinal touch therapy and aromatherapy can be very helpful.

Dietary advice

Follow a detoxing diet.

Other recommendations

- Gentle massage with aromatherapy oils such as marjoram, lavender, juniper, sandalwood and German chamomile can be helpful. Use 1 dessertspoonful almond oil with 3 drops of 2 or 3 oils.

Acupressure points

Gall-bladder 38   This point is found on the outside of the leg, 1 hand and 1 thumb width above the crown of the ankle bone between the shin and the smaller leg bone. Press inwards.

Slipped disc

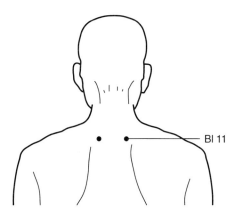

Slipped disc   *Bladder 1 1*

Professional help

Consult your GP or complementary practitioner. See a physiotherapist or osteopath.

Dietary advice

Follow a detoxing diet.

Other recommendations

- Keep the painful area warm.
- Rest as much as possible.

Acupressure points

Bladder 11   This point lies at the top of the ribcage, 2 finger widths from the centre of the spine. Press inwards.

Sports injuries

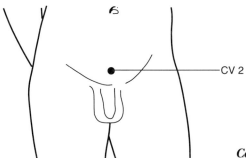

Sprains   *Conception Vessel 2*

Professional help

Consult your GP or complementary practitioner or see a sports physiotherapist.

Dietary advice

Diet is usually not a factor here.

Other recommendations

- A variety of hot or cold compresses may be useful. These can be made with a bowl of hot water and 3 drops lavender, 3 drops marjoram, 3 drops chamomile and 3 drops geranium essential oils.

Acupressure points

- Do not press directly on the site of injury. Select from the chart on pages 40–41 and local points 6 inches or more away from the problem area; use gentle pressure.

Stiffness in general

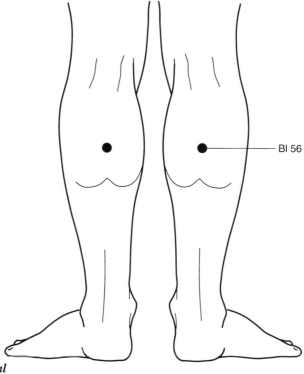

BI 56

Stiffness in general

Bladder 56

Professional help

Consult your GP or complementary practitioner of your choice. Try aromatherapy.

Other recommendations

- A variety of hot or cold compresses may be useful. These can be made with a bowl of hot water and 3 drops lavender, 3 drops marjoram, 3 drops chamomile and 3 drops geranium essential oils.
- Saunas may be helpful.

Acupressure points

Bladder 56   This point is found on the fullest part of the calf muscle, on the centre line. Press firmly inwards.

Sweating (excessive)

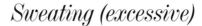
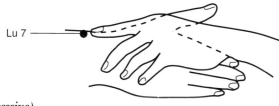

Sweating (excessive)   *Lung 7*

Professional help

Consult your GP or consult a professional acupressurist, acupuncturist or Chinese herbalist.

Dietary advice

Dietary changes may be needed at the discretion of your therapist.

Other recommendations

- Try to keep the body temperature even.
- Avoid draughts.

Acupressure points

Lung 7   This point is found at the thumbside of the hand, 3 thumb widths up from the wristcrease, in line with the thumbnail in the small depression. Press inwards.

Tennis elbow

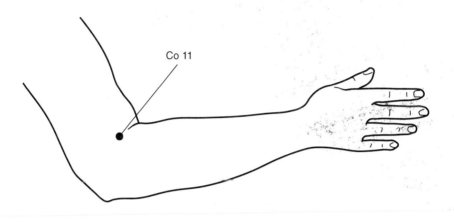

Co 11

Tennis elbow   *Colon 1 1*

Professional help

Consult your GP or physiotherapist. Acupressure can often help.

Dietary advice

Diet is not usually a factor here.

Other recommendations

- Gentle massage with Olbas oil may ease the pain.
- Hot compresses made with a bowl of hot water and 3 drops marjoram, 3 drops peppermint and 3 drops lavender. Apply these at least 3 times a day.
- Avoid over-using or exercising the arm. A sling may be useful while the condition is severe.
- Apply the acupressure point after applying compresses.

Acupressure points

Colon 11   This point lies at the end of the elbow crease, with the arm bent. Press down towards the funny bone.
Colon 15   This point is found in the depression between the top of the arm and the collarbone, at the top of the shoulder, towards the front. Press in and towards the top of the arm (see arthritis of the shoulder).

Tiredness

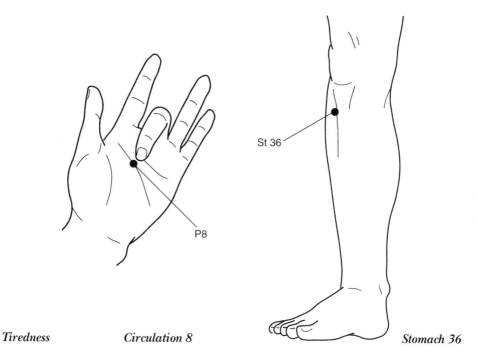

| Tiredness | Circulation 8 | Stomach 36 |

Professional help

Consult your GP if you do not respond to rest and extra sleep.

Dietary advice

A well-balanced diet with plenty of vegetables is essential. Avoid excess tea, coffee, alcohol and sugar. A multi-vitamin complex may be needed for a while.

Other recommendations

- Review your lifestyle and try to change any stress or work overload.
- Relaxing baths may be taken with 2–4 drops of oils such as German chamomile, lavender, geranium and rose.

Acupressure points

Stomach 36   This point is found 3 finger widths under the kneecap, in the hollow on the *outer edge* of the shin. Press inwards.
Pericardium 8   This point is found in the centre of the palm of the hand, where the middle finger rests when folded inwards.

Voice problems

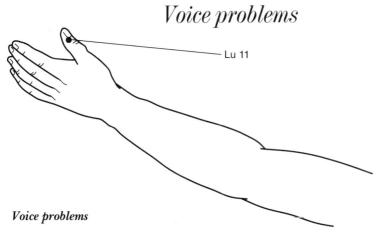

Lu 11

Voice problems   *Lung 11*

Professional help

Consult your GP if the problem is persistent.

Dietary advice

If the problem is caused by chills, go on a cleansing detoxing diet for a few days and increase the intake of fruit and vegetables.

Other recommendations

- Voice problems can sometimes be caused by stress. If this is the case, practise relaxation and meditation techniques.

- If the problem is caused by chills, have drinks of hot water with lemon and honey. Avoid smoking and smoky and over-dry atmospheres.

- Rest the voice, until the symptoms have subsided.

Acupressure points

Lung 11   This point lies at the bottom corner of the nail on the outer side of the thumb. Press vertically inwards.

Treatments during pregnancy
Caution   During the first three months of pregnancy it is important *not* to use aromatherapy oils, other than under the guidance of a qualified aromatherapist. After the third month it is safe to use oils such as rose, neroli, jasmin, sandalwood, lavender and geranium. Use these oils well diluted, for example, 1 dessertspoonful almond oil with 1 drop rose and 3 drops lavender or 1 dessertspoonful almond oil with 1 drop jasmin and 3 drops geranium.

For further advice, see your nearest qualified aromatherapist.

6

SELF-TREATMENT: PREVENTIVE ACUPRESSURE

The best way to start a self-treatment programme is by using preventive methods. A very effective form of this is the Japanese Do-In or Tao-Yinn, the regenerative healing exercises designed to regain hearing of the voice of Nature.

Before beginning these exercises, make sure that you are wearing loose clothing. Find a peaceful space and take a few moments to centre yourself by focusing on your breathing, gradually bringing golden light and energy in with the breath and sending it down to your fingertips.

Head and neck

- Pull as many faces as possible in all directions, especially opening the mouth and eyes very wide. Briskly tap the face with the fingertips of both hands on completion. This improves the blood supply to the skin and exercises the facial muscles, as well as affecting several meridians. Drum gently with loose fists all over the scalp.

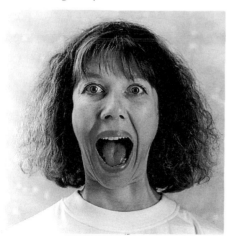 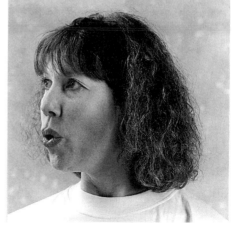

- Using fingers and thumbs, pinch the jawbone from chin to ear with both hands.

- Pinch and pull fleshy part of eyebrows, work from nose to outer corner.

- Massage all round and behind ears, above ear lobes; pinch and pull earlobes. There are acupoints from all meridians on the ears. Ear acupuncture is an independent specialised science.

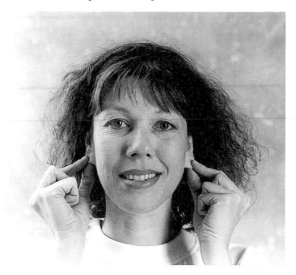

- Place left hand on right, so that the heels of the hands rest either side of the neck, knead and massage up and down the neck. Change hands and work until relaxation is felt. Excellent for neck tension; also stimulates bladder and gall-bladder meridians.

- Spread fingers on scalp with thumbs tucked under the base of the skull; massage deeply along the whole area. Same benefits as neck massage, but with a stronger effect.

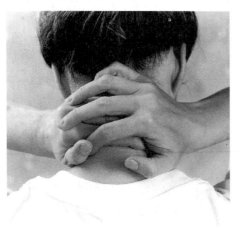
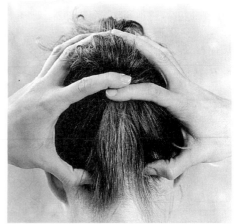

Back – shoulder-blade loosener

This treatment clears tension, protein deposits and benefits the bladder meridian.

- Sitting with a straight spine, relax the right arm and let it swing back.

- Press with stiffened fingertips of the left hand in and along resulting hollow space inside the shoulder blade; massage well all round.

- Finish with a forceful breath through the mouth, as if releasing the 'rubbish' that you have brought to the surface.

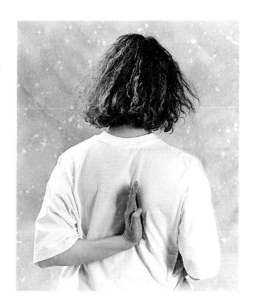

Back – back stimulator

This treatment energises the spine and circulation of the back; it benefits the sciatic nerve, and throat and chest problems.

- Make loose fists and beat up and down each side of the spine with the back of the fists. Use rhythmical movements.

- Breathe out as before.

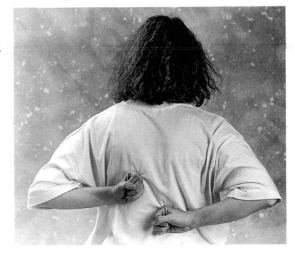

Back – sacral rub

This treatment helps to warm up the kidneys and improve their overall function, as well as general mobility of the lower back.

- With the palms of both hands lying flat on either side of the spine on the lower back, massage up and down until the area becomes very warm.

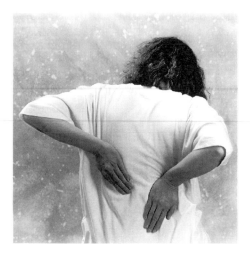

Abdomen

- Lie flat on the floor with the knees bent, and the soles of both feet flat on the floor. Relax the abdomen, place left hand on stomach above the navel and right hand below. Move both hands horizontally back and forth, working in opposite directions.

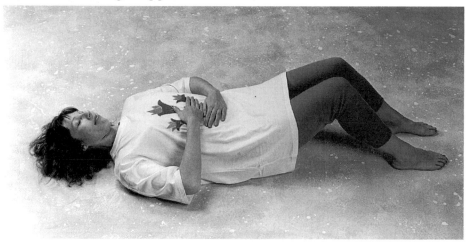

- Fold the hands on top of each other, directly over the navel. Inhale and hold the breath, while circling clockwise with both hands, using firm pressure. Make seven circles, then exhale forcibly through the mouth.

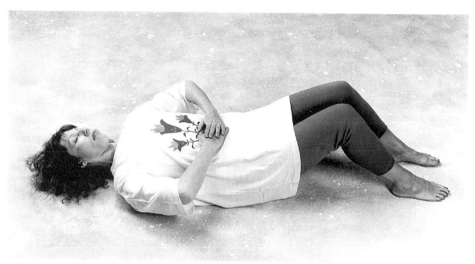

- Inhale. Place the palms of both hands on the belly, just above the thighs. Massage up and down ten times. Exhale all the time. Put more pressure on the up-stroke. This will improve the functioning of food assimilation and elimination.

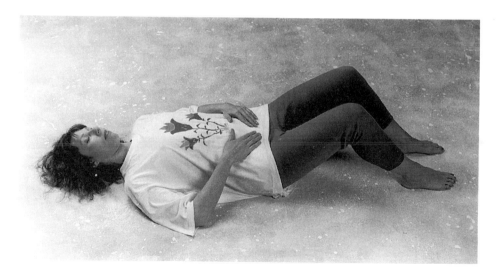

Hands and feet

- Bend wrists backwards and forwards. If a right angle is achieved easily, it indicates good health.

- Flex fingers backwards and fowards, like an oriental dancer.

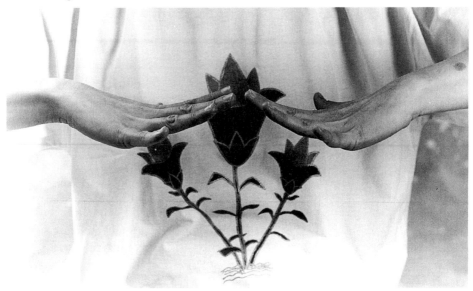

- Press fingers and thumbs (not palms) of both hands together a number of times; this is said to aid the discharge of toxins.

- Massage, rotate and pull fingers and thumbs of both hands; this improves the flow of qi in the six meridians (lung, large intestine, triple heater, pericardium, heart and small intestine).

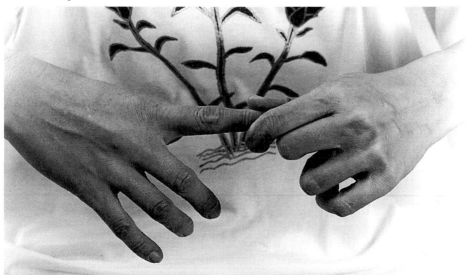

- Lift each foot in turn, rotate slowly clockwise, then anticlockwise, a number of times; shake the feet side to side from the ankle, while exhaling. This is said to be helpful for varicose veins.

- Massage, rotate, pull and pinch each of the toes in turn; this stimulates the flow of qi in six meridians (kidney, spleen, liver, stomach, gall-bladder and bladder). Massage the sole of the foot deeply. Exhale.

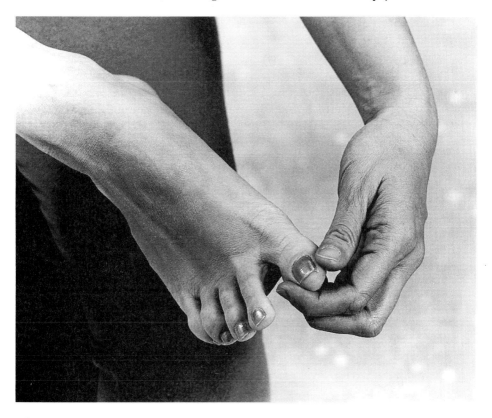

The greatest benefit will be experienced if these exercises are repeated several times a week.

7

PULSE TAKING AND BALANCING POINTS

A major diagnostic tool of oriental medicine is pulse taking. In the West the doctor takes the pulse in just one position and is usually only looking for one thing, the speed of the pulse.

In oriental medicine, a fully trained practitioner can distinguish 28 different qualities of pulse and understand their significance, according to the system called the 'Eight Principal Patterns of Disharmony'. One of the ways these pulses is taken, at a simple level, is by feeling the quality, speed, width, depth, strength and weakness at three positions on each wrist. These different qualities are felt first with light pressure and then with deeper pressure. Each position, light or deep, corresponds to a particular meridian and organ.

PULSE POSITIONS

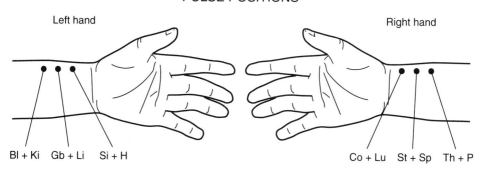

Left hand   Right hand

Bl + Ki   Gb + Li   Si + H   Co + Lu   St + Sp   Th + P

Left hand		Right hand	
Light position	*Deep position*	*Light position*	*Deep position*
Si (Small intestine)	H (Heart)	Co (Colon)	Lu (Lung)
Gb (Gall-bladder)	Lv (Liver)	St (Stomach)	Sp (Spleen)
Bl (Bladder)	Ki (Kidney)	Th (Triple heater)	P (Pericardium)

We can learn to feel whether there is a strong (also called 'full') or a weak (or 'empty') pulse on each of the positions and use one of the appropriate 'source' or 'balancing' points to bring that meridian and the organ it influences back into harmony with the whole system.

Pulse taking is an art that takes a number of years to master. Practise on yourself, then ask friends and family if you can feel their pulse. A 'full' pulse feels strong under the fingers and may push up through the skin. An 'empty' pulse may feel narrow, weak or hardly there.

Pulse taking, Chinese style

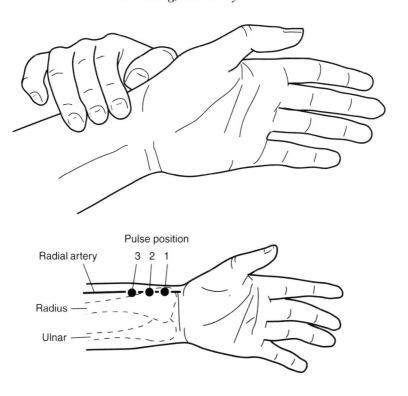

Source points or balancing points

These are points which, when stimulated, have the effect of adjusting the energy in the meridian on which they are located. Source points may be used for either tonification or sedation, depending on the direction of treatment – clockwise tonifies, anticlockwise sedates – or, in acupuncture, the type of needles used and the way the needles are manipulated.

Whatever way the source point is stimulated, it has the effect of automatically re-establishing the balance of energy in the meridian, and, usually, has that effect very rapidly. In other words, the source points can be used, whether the meridian is excessive or deficient, and in either case, they will help to balance the flow.

List of balancing points for each meridian

Lung	(Lu)	9	metal element
Colon	(Co)	4	metal element
Stomach	(St)	42	earth element
Spleen	(Sp)	3	earth element
Triple heater	(Th)	4	fire element
Pericardium	(P)	1	fire element
Small intestine	(Si)	4	fire element
Heart	(H)	7	fire element
Gall-bladder	(Gb)	40	wood element
Liver	(Lv)	3	wood element
Bladder	(Bl)	64	water element
Kidney	(Ki)	3	water element

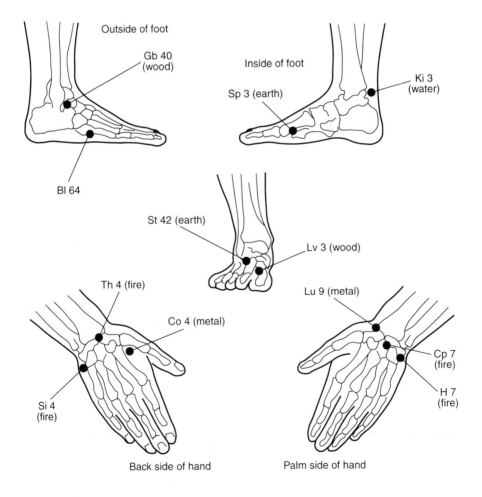

Outside of foot
Gb 40 (wood)
Bl 64

Inside of foot
Ki 3 (water)
Sp 3 (earth)

St 42 (earth)
Lv 3 (wood)

Th 4 (fire)
Co 4 (metal)
Si 4 (fire)
Back side of hand

Lu 9 (metal)
Cp 7 (fire)
H 7 (fire)
Palm side of hand

Point positions

Lung 9 is found in the inner wrist crease, under the base of the thumb. Press firmly inwards.

Colon 4 is found at the end of the crease in the web between the finger and the thumb. Press towards the fingerbone on the hand.

Stomach 42 is found centrally, 2 fingers width down from the ankle crease on the top of the foot. Press inwards.

Spleen 3 lies about half an inch above the big toe joint on the side of the bone. Press inwards.

Triple heater 4 lies on the back of the wrist centrally on the wrist crease. Press inwards.

Pericardium 1 is found centrally on the crease of the inner wrist. Press inwards.

Small intestine 4 lies at the side of the hand in a depression about three quarters of an inch above the wrist in line with the little finger. Press inwards.

Heart 7 is found on the inner wrist crease, directly in line with the little finger. Press inwards.

Gallbladder 40 lies in the depression under the outer ankle bone towards the top of the foot. Press towards the centre of the foot.

Liver 3 lies in the web between the big toe and the next toe. Press in and up towards the centre of the foot.

Bladder 64 is found on the outside of the foot on the upper slopes of the largest bone, coming up from the little toe, before it becomes the heel. Press inwards.

Kidney 3 is found in the hollow between the inner ankle bone and the Achilles tendon. Press firmly inwards.

General self-balancing treatment

Ideally, the general self-balancing treatment given here should be carried out at least once a month, to maintain optimum health, strengthen the nervous system, and counteract the stresses and strains of daily life.

The treatment can also be used to great advantage in conjunction with, or prior to, other treatments, for example the first aid treatment described in Chapter 5. It can be very helpful for people who have to endure a period of enforced inactivity, such as a result of a broken leg, as it keeps the energy moving throughout the body, and through the spine, which is particularly important. Used as a preliminary to meditation, the treatment will have a quietening effect and bring an inner calm. The treatment can also be adapted for use by couples.

The Central Channel, which is the Governing Vessel at the back and the Conception Vessel at the front, is one continuous flow of fundamental energy. Since it is the most powerful meridian it has a strong effect on the body, mind and emotions. This self-treatment pattern makes use of several beneficial acupoints along this channel. It is better done lying down, but may be done in a sitting position. Use fingertips and palms of hands.

GV.1   Stabilises and energises. Calms the mind.

CV.2   Calms the belly and strengthens the reproductive system and bladder.

CV.12   Warms and energises the stomach and spleen. Improves appetite. Also for tiredness, tension and anxiety.

CV.17   (Centre of breast bone, between nipples) Clears tightness in the chest, stimulates breathing and relaxes the diaphragm.

GV.24.5   Calms the mind.

GV.20   (Centrally, top of head, just as it begins to slope down at back) Clears the mind and lifts the spirits.

GV.15   Effective for severe anxiety, relaxes the base of the skull and inhibits headaches.

Other points

GB.14   (Between hairline and eyebrow, centrally above pupils) Relaxes and calms the mind, eases frontal headaches.

St.15   (One rib space above halfway line between nipples and collarbone) Calming and refreshing and aids deep breathing.

LV.12   Improves liver and bowel function.

Points and areas in order of use

STEP 1   1   Right hand – CV 2 and left hand – CV 12
             2   Palms over LV 12 with fingertips touching CV 2
             3   Move left hand CV 17 and leave right hand

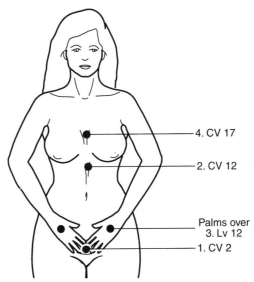

Part 1 - General balancing self– treatment

STEP 2   1   Left hand – GV 15 and right hand – GV 1

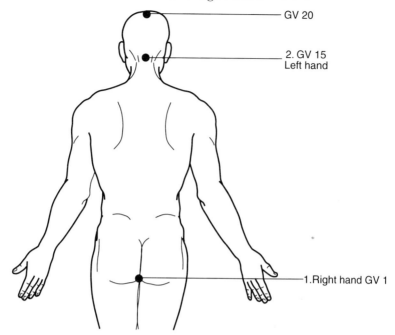

Part 2

STEP 3   1   Palms over St 15
           2   Left hand GV 20 and right hand – GV 24.5 (third eye)
           3   Fingers over GB 14 with tips touching GV 24.5

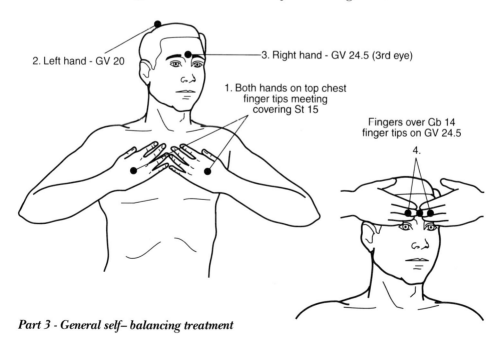

Part 3 - General self– balancing treatment

STEP 4   1   Left hand GV 19 and right hand – GV 1

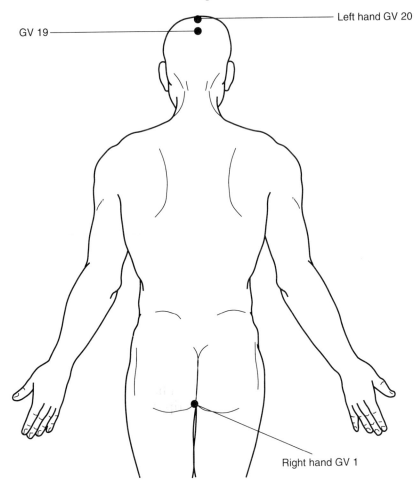

Part 4 - Self– treatment general self– balancing

New points that are given in this treatment are:

Conception vessel (CV) 17; Stomach (St) 15; Governing Vessel (GV) 20; Gall-bladder (Gb) 14

Self-help treatment chart

You should by now be feeling confident enough to embark on regular self-treatment. To encourage you and help you to keep track of your progress, we have included a self-help treatment chart in the Appendix (pages 108–109). We have made this photocopiable so that you may keep a record of each new problem you decide to try to overcome. Good luck!

8

ACUPRESSURE FOR SPECIAL SITUATIONS

Office stress

This treatment alleviates 'office stress', insomnia, hangovers, and toxic build up due to too much rich or acidic food. It is given at the end of every Shen Tao treatment to make sure that the qi is flowing properly round the head and neck; you can also try it yourself.

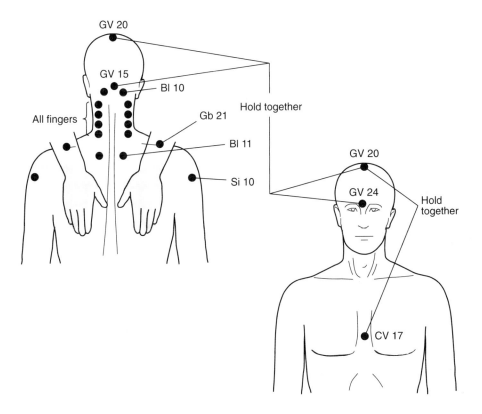

Lie on your back with your elbows propped up by pillows. Breathe in 'Light and Energy' and send this through the fingertips. You can treat a friend if you wish. Stand behind your friend and insert step 2.

1 Si 10
Fold the palm of your hand around the top of your shoulder (as if holding a tennis ball), and rest the fingertip of the middle finger at the back (the finger should automatically tuck under the rounded bone and fall into a slight dip).

2 Si 11
(This step is only necessary if you are treating someone else.) Slide your hands under the shoulder blades (which feel like an upside down triangle), and hold palms over Si 11 (use your intuitive feeling and let your hands guide you to the right spot; do not forget that there is a lot of strength in maintaining a flow of awareness).

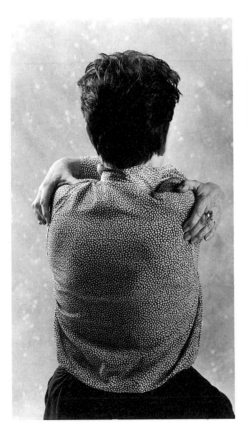 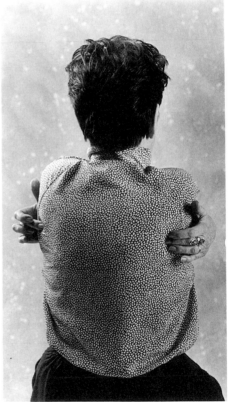

3 Bl 11

Bring the fingertips of the middle fingers up to Bl 11. Bl 11 is found on either side of the spine, about two finger widths from the centre line of the spine, level with the top of the shoulder blade.

4 Gb 21

Move the fingertips up the shoulders to Gb 21, which is found at the highest point of the shoulder, as shown in the photograph.

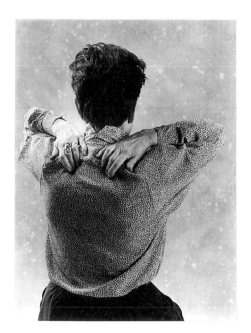

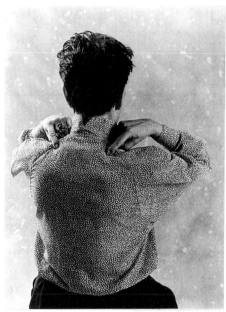

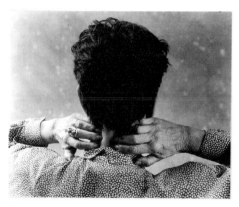

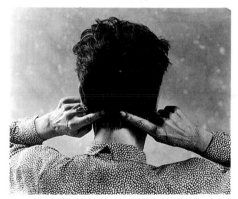

5 Bl X

Hold the fingertips of index, middle, ring, and little finger gently alongside the cervical vertebrae (*not* on the vertebrae itself).

6 Bl 10

Both sides of the neck under the skull are activated simultaneously with the fingers.

7 GV 20 AND GV 15
Now hold one fingertip on GV 15 and the fingertip of the other hand at the top of the head on GV 20.

8 Keep the palm of one hand over GV 20, and move the other hand to CV 17, which is the point lying on the breastbone, between the nipples of both breasts.

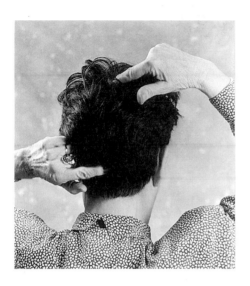
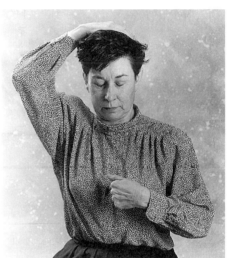

Harmonising treatment for use by couples

This treatment may be done with or without clothing, whichever feels the most comfortable. For couples, the treatment could be combined with essential oils, such as 1 drop rose, 4 drops geranium and 4 drops bergamot in 1 dessertspoonful almond oil. The points could then be included as part of a sensuous and relaxing massage.

The points used in this pattern are designed to bring a feeling of relief from stress and tension, and a general sensation of well-being.

POINTS USED

1   GB 21   Brings relief to overburdened shoulders, a place where many people hold a lot of tension. Benefits the gall-bladder, liver and digestive system.

2   Ki 1   Eases the feet, brings a feeling of letting-go, going with flow.

3   GV 4   Brings relief from lower back and kidney problems, aches and pains from too much sitting. Brings warmth to the feminine side of the body (yin) and nourishes the reproductive system.

	CV 8&6	Energising and warming, helps the digestive system. Brings the qi to the masculine side of the body (yang).
4	GV 1	Brings a feeling of grounding and stabilisation.
	Bl 62	Brings a feeling of relaxation and calmness, as well as clarity of the mind. Good for those who worry and tend to have a lack of concentration.
5	St 36	Major tonic point for whole body, also warms and energises the stomach, improves digestion and assimilation of food.
6	Si 10	Calming point for the mind. When holding this point some past memories may come up; keep holding this point until any disturbances are cleared.
	Th 5 & P 6	Releasing nervous tension, as well as emotional holding. Calms the spirit.

STEP	POSITION	POINT
1	Stand (or kneel) at top of head both hands on shoulders	palms on Gb 21
2	Stand (or kneel) at feet	both thumbs on Ki 1
3	Stand (or kneel) at *right* side of partner; slide *left* hand under the back at waist level	palm covers GV 4
	& *right* hand on front at waist level	palm over CV 8 (belly button) + CV 6
4	*Left* hand slides down to tip of coccyx	palm covers GV 1
	& *right* hand to outside ankle	tip finger on Bl 62
5	*Left* hand stays	on GV 1
	& *right* hand below knee	tip finger on St 36
6	*Left* hand to top arm	tip finger on Si 10
	& *right* hand around wrist	using tip middle finger on Th 5 (top of wrist) and tip thumb on P 6 (on inside wrist)

Complete with Neck and Shoulder Relaxing Treatment

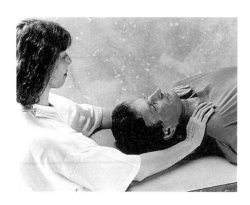

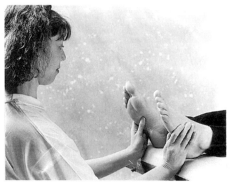

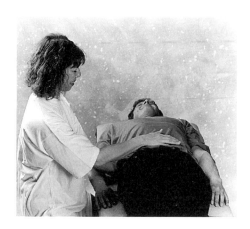

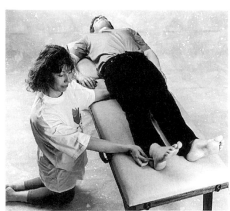

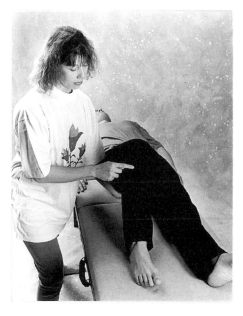

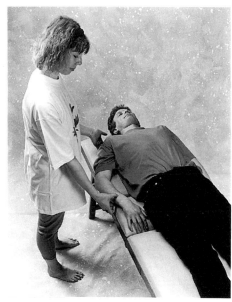

Effective acupressure facial

Spend five minutes a day on this simple routine to improve the circulation, relax stress and tension in the face, ward off headaches and 'thick heads' and clear nasal congestion.

Massage each point clockwise for 30 seconds in the following order.

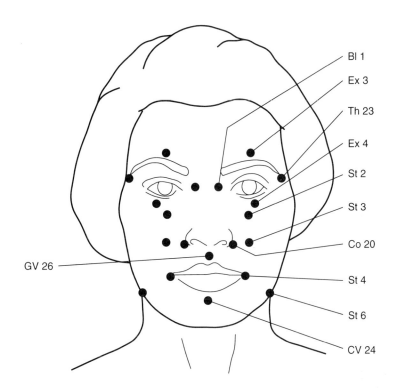

The specific properties of each point are as follows:

Bl 1	eye conditions
St 2	tired eyes, twitching
Ex 4	said to improve short sight
Th 23	headaches, eye conditions
Ex 3	tones facial muscles, helps eye problems
GV 26	shock and heat stroke
Co 20	sinusitis, colds
St 3	pain and swelling of lips, cheeks, toothache
St 4	relaxes over-taut facial muscles
St 6	toothache and muscular spasm
GV 24	swelling gums and toothache

9

WHAT TO EXPECT FROM AN ACUPRESSURE TREATMENT

With the professional forms of acupressure that work with both hands and give a full body treatment (Shen Tao, Jin Shin Do, Jin Shin Jyitsu and Shiatsu), profound relaxing and re-energising effects will be noticed, sometimes lasting for a number of weeks. The usual benefits to health and well-being include sounder sleep, a general feeling of relaxation (both physical and mental), more energy and enthusiasm for life and the steady improvement of the initial problem, especially if the technique is combined with a healthier diet and sufficient rest and exercise.

Possible short-term effects

However, healing usually includes cleansing and clearing of the system, having been stimulated by the treatment. This may take the form of headaches, expelling of mucus, or aches and pains. These are the body's ways of releasing toxins. This can also apply to unexpressed emotional pain, such as grief or shock, which becomes a damaging energy if held too long within the cells of the body, and can lower our resistance and deplete the immune system. In clearing toxins and negative emotion, acupressure gently strengthens the system and helps rejuvenate and promote a sense of relaxation and well-being.

It is essential to rest after an acupressure treatment, ideally for the same length of time that the treatment lasted. This allows the subtle shifts and re-alignment of energy to take place in a very natural way.

This is espcially true of Shen Tao, where patterns of energy or vibrational frequencies are built up, rather like a piece of music when more notes are being added to the original composition. Many people experience this as something like the sound frequencies of music, others report wave sensations of warmth and moving tingling energy, and always feel profound relaxation by the end of the treatment. The benefits of acupressure are usually felt very rapidly. As the immune system gains strength and the flow of life-giving qi is restored to every particle, the organs and body systems heal and regenerate, and the effects of imbalances clear up. The speed of this healing will depend on the age, constitution, amount of vitality and mental attitude of the recipient.

Long-term benefits

Self-treament is ideal as preventive medicine and optimum health maintenance, however, if specific problems do occur and fail to respond to self-treatment after a few weeks, then it is time to consult a health-care professional. Chronic problems already being treated by orthodox means will often be greatly improved by the additional use of self-treatment acupressure on a daily basis.

Acupressure is also an excellent way of restoring full health after a debilitating illness, operation, childbirth, or any period of severe mental, emotional or physical stress. Children respond well to acupressure, as do elderly people and those who find the thought of needles quite unacceptable. The benefits of oriental medicine are still available to them through these different forms of touch therapy.

A typical professional treatment

A professional treatment may, in the case of Shen Tao, for example, go as follows.

The client will be welcomed and a detailed case history will be taken, which explores not only medical history, but the kind of emotional climate that the client grew up in and the various stresses and strains currently being experienced. For Shen Tao, light clothing is worn and the client relaxes on his/her back on a comfortable couch and is not required to turn or move around. The practitioner will then take a pulse reading from both wrists and probably use a tongue diagnosis as well. (The tongue is a sensitive instrument which reveals the state of health and the imbalances within the meridian system. The experienced practitioner will look at the shape and colour of the tongue and its superficial 'fur'. Dryness and moistness also contribute to the diagnosis.)

Together with the information from the consultation, a choice is made of treatment patterns, usually using one of the 'extra meridians', followed by one or two meridian patterns, and finally fine-tuning with single points. The treatment is always completed with a neck relaxing pattern. Fingertips of both hands are used, creating an energy circuit with the client, and the breathing in of 'Light and Healing' is directed through the fingers to the client. The pulses are checked again to register the changes that have taken place.

It is advisable to rest for up to an hour after each treatment, if possible.

Flower remedies

Chinese herbs are often prescribed with traditional acupuncture. However, with the sensitive form of acupressure, known as Shen Tao, it has been found that the Bach and other flower remedies, which are taken by mouth, form the perfect combination with their gentle, yet profound, effect. Flower remedies have an ability to bring healing to emotional and mental imbalances and, in this way, affect the whole body. Clients may be encouraged to choose their own remedies and it is often noticed that they choose those remedies that are immediately needed. If the client continues for some months having further consultations, it is often noticed that they then choose to go to a more profound level of healing with the next remedy. It can be compared to the peeling of an onion; each time another layer is taken off, it allows healing to reach a deeper level. Changes are usually noticed after a few weeks, but sometimes only after some months.

The flower remedies are excellent, because they are very gentle in their way of working with the person as a whole; they are non-intrusive, yet they have a profound effect on the physical and emotional being.

APPENDIX

Repertoire of additional applications for the points

Lu
1   asthma, breathing difficulties, strengthens chest tension, congestion.
9   asthma and coughing.
11   tonsillitis, fever, epilepsy, coma, respiratory failure.

Co
4   frontal headaches, shoulder pain
11   constipation and indigestion, reduces feverish colds, arthritic elbow pain, helps intestines and immune system.

15   frozen shoulders, pain and stiffness of elbow and arm.
20   clears sinus, facial swelling, nasal congestion.

St
4   saliva deficiency, facial paralysis, neuralgia.
15   bronchitis, asthma, distention and pain in chest.
35   rheumatism of feet and *oedema* (swelling caused by water retention), knee pain.
36   whole body tonic, especially for muscles, helps dizziness and exhaustion.

Sp
6   water retention, diarrhoea, regulates menstruation and balances reproductive system.

Th
5   deafness, headache, tinnitus.

P
6   indigestion, sea sickness and morning sickness, insomnia, nervous palpitations.

Si
19   eye complaints, headaches.

Gb

20   migraine, headaches, dizziness, stiff neck, eye strain, arthritis.

30   helps tendons and stiff joints, hip pain, rheumatism (localised).

34   sciatica, knee pain, muscular problems, relaxes muscles in lower body.

40   sciatica, shoulder pain and headaches, twisted ankles.

Lv

12   relieves stomachache, diarrhoea, nausea, headaches.

3   allergic reactions, headaches, hangovers, tired eyes, foot cramps.

Bl

2   sinus pain, eye pain, hay fever, hangovers.

10   insomnia, exhaustion, stiff neck.

11   aching shoulder joint, fever, cough.

40   knee joint pain, back pain, sciatica.

56   leg pain, stiffness and pain in back and lumbar region, haemorrhoids.

58   cystitis, legs weak and painful.

62   headache, dizziness, epilepsy.

Ki

1   stimulates kidneys, hot flushes, helps impotence, epilepsy.

3   tinnitus, earache, fatigue, swollen feet, insomnia, helps immune and reproductive system.

6   reproductive problems, swelling and painful ankles, insomnia.

Pregnancy and childbirth

CV 6   (See self-treatment chart on pages 40–41 for position of point) Infertility.

P 6   (See self-treatment chart on pages 40–41) Indigestion and morning sickness.

Co 4   (See self-treatment chart on pages 40–41) *Not* for pregnant women, as may stimulate contraction of uterus, but will help labour pains.

Bl 67   (Close to outside of nail of little toe) Difficult labour.

Ki 3   (See self-treatment chart on pages 40–41) *Not* for pregnant women, but will help difficult labour; helps reproductive and immune system.

ST 16   (On nipple line, vertically halfway up, between nipple and collarbone, one rib space under ST 15. See general self-balancing treatment on page 89) Breast pain; aids lactation.

Sp 6   Regulates menstrual cycle and balances reproductive system.

Emotions

Fear and anxiety	Bl 40; Ki 1; GV 26
Worry and stress	hold big toe, affects spleen and liver
	Bl 62 (for calm sleeping) Co 11 CV 24.5 P 6
Anger	P 9 (tip of middle finger) Lv 3 Gb 40, 30, 20 Lv 9
Grief, as well as inability to grieve	Lu 1 Lu 9 (base of thumb) CV 17
Depression	H 9 (tip of little finger) Co 4 Bl 10 GV 20 CV 17

Self-help treatment chart

Date: ....

LIST PROBLEM AREAS AND MARK
ON BODY CHART

....

....

NOTE DOWN MENTAL OR
EMOTIONAL STRESS

....

....

Record your pulses in the
following way:

V = normal / + = full or fast
– = empty, weak or slow

PULSE CHART

Left Hand		Right Hand	
Si		Li	Lu
Gb		St	Sp
Ki		Th	P
LIGHT	DEEP	LIGHT	DEEP
	H		
	Lv		
	Bl		

I have chosen to activate the following points

....

....

(mark these also on the body chart above).

I shall treat myself regularly for .... number of days; .... weeks

Note any situations that make my condition worse: ....

....

Describe the changes you have noticed after:

4 days ....

1 week ....

3 weeks ....

Notice especially changes in your pulse and general feeling of well-being and energy, plus diminishment of tension, both physical and mental.

Date: ....

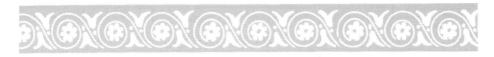

FURTHER READING

Bek, Lilla and Pullar, Phillipa, *7 Levels of Healing*, Century Hutchinson Ltd, 1986

De Langre, Jacques, *Do In*, Happiness Press, 1978

Harvey, Clare and Cochrane, Amanda, *The Encyclopaedia of Flower Essences*, Thorsons, February 1995

Kaptchuk, Ted, *Chinese Medicine: The Web That Has No Weaver*, Rider, 1983

Kennet, Roshi Jiyu and McPhillamy, Rev. Daizu, *The Book of Life*, Shasta Abbey Press, 1979

Motoyama, Hiroshi, *Theories of the Chakras*, Theosophical Publishing House, 1981

Oki, Masahiro, *Zen Yoga Therapy*, Japan Publications Inc, 1979

Soo, Chee, *Tao of Long Life*, Gordon & Cremonesi, 1979

Soo, Chee, *The Taoist Ways of Healing*, Aquarian Press, 1986

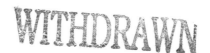

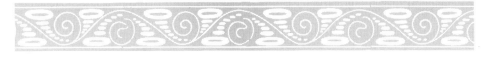

USEFUL ADDRESSES

The Acupressure Institute
1533 Shattuck Avenue
Berkley
California 94709 USA
(Tel: 808 442 2232)

The Shiatsu Society
14 Oakdene Road
Redhill
Surrey
RH1 6BT
(Tel: 0737 767896)

Jin Shin Jyutsu
8719 E. San Alberto
Scottsdale
Arizona 85258
USA

The Shen Tao Association
Middle Piccadilly Natural Healing
  Centre
Holwell, Nr Sherborne
Dorset DT9 5LW
(Tel: 0963 23468)
Send s.a.e. for practitioner list.